100 WAYS TO A HEALTHY 100

Simple Steps to Health, Longevity and Youthfulness

Deborah Peden

100 Ways To A Healthy 100
Simple Secrets to Health, Longevity and Youthfulness

First published in Australia by A New Pinnacle Life Coaching 2019
www.100waystoahealthy100.com.au
www.anewpinnaclelifecoaching.com.au

Copyright © Deborah Peden 2019
All Rights Reserved

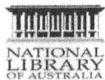

A catalogue record for this book is available from the National Library of Australia

ISBN: 978-0-6485320-0-2 (pbk)
ISBN: 978-0-6485320-1-9 (ebk)

Typesetting and design by Publicious Book Publishing
Published in collaboration with Publicious Book Publishing
www.publicious.com.au

Illustrations by Sean Leahy © 2019

Disclaimer: This book contains information that is intended to help readers be better informed consumers of health care and wellbeing. It is presented as general advice on health and wellbeing. Always consult a qualified doctor or health professional for your individual needs. The author and publisher do not accept responsibility for illness or injury arising out of the failure to seek medical advice from a doctor. In the event that you use any of the information in this book for yourself or your family and friends, the author and publisher assume no responsibility for your actions.

Why I wrote this book

My purpose is to bring together the knowledge and wisdom of others for whom good health is paramount, and to educate and inspire my readers to optimum wellbeing for a purpose-filled life and for their own betterment and that of our planet.

This book is dedicated to my husband, Don, who has patiently been 'educated' as I subjected him to the knowledge and research for this book.

God has entrusted me with myself—Epictetus.

Foreword, by Dr John Demartini

In a world saturated with information on how to ward off disease, sustain wellness and find the elixir to a long life, there emerges a gem that is worthy of attention. *100 Ways to a Healthy 100* is one of those, and it's come into your hands for a reason. What makes this book unique? The answer lies in its ability to harvest the pearls from a sea of health and wellbeing treasures, transforming the collective wisdom of ancient and contemporary sources into an easy-to-read guide, interspersed with a mix of humor, story and heart-warming analogies.

I first 'met' Deb in a desolate region of Australia. It was about ten years ago when she and a friend shared a drive across the Nullarbor Plain. Her friend's copy of my book, *The Breakthrough Experience*, lay open on the backseat of the car. Intrigued, Deb asked to read it and over the several day journey across this wilderness, she did just that. Inspired by what she read, Deb and I would eventually meet in person when she became a student of mine and then a Demartini Method facilitator assisting me live at my *Breakthrough Experience* seminars.

As a human behavior specialist and educator, I have dedicated over four and a half decades of my life to helping people expand their potential, in order for them to live extraordinary lives. I have learned that the key to exceptional achievement and fulfilment lies in finding out what is most valuable and meaningful to people so they can access their greatness. When this happens, an inspiring leader emerges, one who embraces the voice and vision within themselves, values service to others and the rewards this brings — a form of momentum-building sustainable fair exchange if you will. Deb Peden is an example of one such individual: in researching and writing her book she has been inspired to trust her own potential in order to help others live extraordinary and healthy lives.

The extraordinary aspect of this book is its breadth of knowledge and wisdom on a diverse range of topics, distilled in an easy-to-read manner, and injected with Deb's unique style to inform, entertain and inspire us to reach beyond 100 years of age in vibrant good health.

100 Ways to a Healthy 100 is a worthy read, not just for its information and charm, but because it represents and reflects a fine example of an individual who was inspired to listen to the voice and vision within to convey a message to serve and inspire others.

Dr John F Demartini – International best-selling author of *The Values Factor*

Preface

Two key episodes occurred in my life that were my catalyst for change, and the inspiration for writing this book. The first occurred in September 2008 when I first read the newly published *Sweet Poison* by David Gillespie. The second was an appointment with two physicians. From Gillespie's opening pages, I felt as if the book had been written just for me. And it came into my hands at exactly the right time: I was ready to hear his message, delivered simply yet powerfully, about the toxic effects of sugar in our diet. As a sugar 'addict' I had already known (but didn't want to know) that all that 'good stuff' could be so bad for me. As I turned Gillespie's early pages, I read the history of sugar and how it came to play such a significant role in the 'foods' I purchased from the supermarket. But it was the science explained in layperson's terms of what this substance was doing to me inside and out that was a defining experience.

I was to have confirmation of Gillespie's findings when I came across the research of Dr Robert Lustig the following year. Lustig is a paediatric endocrinologist from the University of California. In his seminal presentation, *Sugar: The Bitter Truth* (2009), which has been viewed online 7.7 million times to date, he demonstrates a scientific mapping of the human body with the consumption of alcohol versus fructose. The result is the same chronic outcome for the liver – minus the head buzz that comes with consuming alcohol. Once I was presented with this *bitter truth* for my lifestyle choices, I just couldn't un-know it.

The second event was a natural consequence of the first. I made two medical appointments, the first to my local doctor for a check-up and some tests. It was probably no surprise to learn that my blood test results returned a 6.7 reading in my blood sugars – not *serious*-serious, but a level considered pre-diabetic. If that news wasn't dismal enough, I sought the advice of a medical doctor specialising in naturopathy. The first thing he did was take my pH reading. I gave him a copy of my blood test results while there.

He picked up on my ALT reading (alanine aminotransferase) of 52, which he translated as an indicator of a fatty liver! He looked grim (bordering on 'cranky' if I'm honest) when reading this result and viewing my pH test result of 4.5, which, he said sternly, was "extremely acidic". A low pH level is an indicator of the oxidation and inflammation my body was harbouring. The numbers didn't look good. Yet, I *looked* healthy, even if I didn't always feel great. And looks can be dangerously deceptive. I was what Dr Lustig would describe as a TOFI (thin on the outside, fat on the inside)! It was a wake-up call and while I had been slow to admit it to that point, something had to change, or I would be living a debilitating life, a short one — or both! We all pay the price for our excesses and indulgences eventually. As Robert Louis Stevenson so aptly put it: "There will come a time when we will sit down to a banquet of our consequences." In reflecting on Stevenson's caution, my intention here is to guide you to a healthier consequence.

Gillespie's book and those medical visits were the beginning of my journey of discovery and yearning to learn more about vibrant good health and how to make it to my hundredth milestone in good nick. My research would confirm that I was already doing much to support my health and wellbeing (sugar addiction aside, of course).

This book is a holistic approach to health, embracing all seven areas of our lives — Mental, Vocational, Physical, Spiritual, Familial, Financial, and Social. I have learned how important it is to take this holistic approach to health in order to reach those golden years hale and hearty.

My experience as a life coach has taught me the value and importance of emotional/psychological good health. I've been privileged to hear stories of challenge as well as triumph. I'm inspired by the courage and persistence that these brave people have demonstrated in overcoming old wounds or current trials by addressing the issues and adopting new ways of perceiving life's challenges. Emotions can be powerful blocks to good health.

Resolving and reconciling the past can clear the path to a longer-living healthier you. As I was once sagely counselled: "You can't change the past, but the past can kill you." Those words shook me at the time. They also moved me to recognise how old emotional wounds were still playing out in the present and that I needed to let them go.

I've included some practical yet powerful strategies here to support emotional wellbeing. There's compelling evidence of the interconnection between our physical and emotional health. Science has made explicit links between the health of our gut (the physical) and our mental wellbeing (our emotions). Known as the gut-brain axis, this theme appears several times among the 100 areas addressed.

Choosing 100 topics seemed like the ideal number when I started writing this book, because of the tidy link to the 100 years I'd wish for all of us living on this planet. Yet many of my readers may well need to do a lot less than I did in order to gain, retain and/or sustain optimum health. I've learned, over my years of previously eating and living in a misguided 'I'm invincible' way, that what might work for me may not necessarily work for others and vice versa. Also, as we move from youth through our more mature years and into our golden years, our needs and circumstances can differ. The figure of 100 gives options for all my readers. Some would argue that we're living longer anyway with advances in medical science. And this is true. However, I'll pose a question that Dr Libby Weaver, one of my favourite authors and a holistic nutrition expert, likes to put forward: 'Are we living too short and dying too long?' (2013a:23). What Weaver implies is the notion that many of our extra years of life may well be spent in a state of ill-health and disease. The holy grail to reaching our centenary and beyond (the 'beyond' folk are known as supercentenarians) is good health (Sachdev, 2013). Research on centenarians has revealed some commonalities among these golden folks: few are obese; they remain physically active across their lifespan; they manage stress well and are adaptable to life's experiences; they're sociable; they do things that give meaning to their lives; and they exercise both their minds and their bodies (Second Opinion, 2016).

There is, of course, the 'gene factor' in which longevity is simply linked to DNA. There are some who will have come from a long ancestral line of folks who have lived long and relatively healthy lives, perhaps despite some poor lifestyle choices. For the rest of us, however, there's the comforting statistic that attributes 30% to good genes and the remaining 70% to lifestyle and environmental factors, for long-life outcomes. While it's natural to die (our bodies inevitably decay, like all mortal creatures), my belief is that it's also natural to live and die disease-free. In fact, it's our birthright to live a healthy life until the day we die. To do this, we initially need to have access to the knowledge, wisdom and opportunity to achieve vibrant, balanced health for at least a century! I'm conscious of the fact that we don't all have equal access to good nutrition, health practitioners and the like. I've tried to keep many of the solutions that will help my readers enjoy a healthy way of life as easy, affordable and accessible as possible. In an ideal world, of course, we'd all be given access to these fundamental rights.

I have another agenda in bringing these 100 healthy tips to you. That agenda centres around my belief that if we live at our optimum then we're providing ourselves with a really solid foundation upon which to make the most of this life and fulfil our purpose for being here – whatever that might be. In essence, my thinking is that we'll be able to maximise our lives and our reason for being, if we can do it from a platform of peak performance. And that, I believe, can be obtained through good health in all its forms.

In compiling these 100 topics, I have drawn on the seven key areas of life, as mentioned above. The idea behind this approach is to provide a healthy balance across our lives. While the concept of health takes many forms, I do, nevertheless, underpin my writing with the philosophy of 'we are what we eat', so you may find I give attention to the foods to eat and those to avoid. Hippocrates, the father of medicine, has been heavily influential. This wise ancient stated: *Let Food be thy Medicine, and Medicine thy Food.*

You'll find that the topics vary in length and theme – some are extensive, others relatively brief. That's because some elements of our health and lifestyle choices require more explanation than others. And, to be honest, I've also included the subjects I'm most passionate about and so I elaborate a little more on those. Where possible, I've included stories to demonstrate the efficacy of particular topics on health. Narrative is not only an entertaining way to make a point, but also a powerful teacher for us. I love learning from others and I'm inspired by the examples they set.

Almost daily I hear or read in the media of miracle medicines, magic potions and quick-fixes that will help us shed excess weight, slow down the aging process or prevent all manner of debilitating and life-threatening diseases. While we await the outcome of such cure-alls, what I offer now are long-term lifestyle changes you can make to turn your health around and give you much greater odds for skipping your way to your hundredth birthday and beyond. Perhaps what follows may well be the natural elixir of youth you've been looking for. If you'd like to use these strategies to attain or regain good health and set a goal, then may I suggest you set yourself a 12-month goal but break it down into weekly sub-goals. If you applied two or three of these ideas each week, then you'd have addressed all areas of your health and lifestyle within the 12 months. I would caution you, however, to first check in with a health professional before modifying your health regime, and especially so if you have any concerns about your health or have a current health condition.

So, let's begin our journey of 100 ways to a healthy 100...

Table of Contents

1. Get raw and real

When I was a kid, the standard fare at the dinner table was 'meat and three veg', the 'veg' typically being peas, beans and potatoes, but occasionally there'd be cauliflower, broccoli or other greens. Any kid worth their salt who wanted to avoid their vegetables needed to be resourceful if they wanted to produce an empty plate without having actually consumed the veggies. With no family dog under the table to save the day, and no sci-fi dematerialisation or teleportation process likely, there was little hope of getting around eating them. Eventually, it was the command to 'eat your veggies or there'll be no pudding' from the adult division of the dinner table that did the trick.

Time has moved on, and I've changed. I've come to my senses and discovered the delicious wonder of the plant-based world, from the unassuming artichoke to the zesty zucchini, all without the need for sugary inducements. No longer averse, I became a raw and real food convert. My 'raw and real' reference is meant to stand in contrast to its evil nemesis: processed foods. If your 'food' (I use this term very loosely here) comes in a box or a packet and has a list of ingredients on its wrapping, then it's processed and will more than likely contain some ingredients that you won't recognise as food. That's because they're not food; they're chemicals. Even many of our breads are highly processed, containing chemicals, added sugars, preservatives, and food colouring to make them look brown and wholesome.

If you want to live a long and healthy life, the idea is to eat as low down the food chain as possible. So says gerontologist and researcher of *The Okinawan Project*, Dr Craig Willcox (2009). Real food comes in its natural state, without preservatives or additives, and can either be eaten raw or cooked depending on the food. Examples of real food are fresh fruit and vegetables, dairy products such as organic yoghurt, milk and cheese, nuts, red meat, fish, and white meats such as chicken and turkey.

A Harvard study found that eating primarily plant-based proteins over processed meats such as sausages and hot dogs equated to a lower risk of death, especially from heart-disease-related illnesses. In fact, for every 3% increase in plant protein you consume, you're reducing your risk of death by 10%. This is because plant-based proteins supply the nine amino acids that our bodies can't produce on their own. They help to lower blood pressure, reduce the risk of heart disease and decrease cancer. Plant-based proteins can be sourced from spinach, potatoes, lentils, sundried tomatoes, peas, soybeans, a range of seeds, and nuts and quinoa, among others (Donvito, 2018). If you're contemplating processed over real/raw food, keep in mind this wise maxim from genetic epidemiologist, Professor Tim Spector: "If your great-grandmother wouldn't recognize it as food, don't eat it" (Spector, 2016). And if you needed one, a final reason for eating raw and real is that you reduce your carbon footprint when you opt for plant-based and other real foods over processed foods (Marie, 2016). For the environmentalists among us, the packaging element alone is a big persuader.

2. Get to know your local greengrocer

Getting to know your greengrocer will help you choose some of the best raw and real food available. It's a much better shopping experience than trundling down supermarket aisles with their abundance of processed foods. Or, you could go one step further and find out where your nearest organic farmer's market is and shop there. My fruit and veg supplier is conveniently located only a few hundred metres from my home. They purchase their supplies from the markets about three times a week, so freshness is their motto. They'll always let me know what's fresh and what's best. I'm really into reading about superfoods at the moment, so my greengrocer has inspired me to eat purple carrots and lots of kale and spinach. Step aside, Popeye! And if you were never a fan of broccoli as a kid, as an adult you might now be excited to learn that it's not only high in vitamin C but that it may also help type 2 diabetes sufferers, according to a recent study (Axelsson *et al* 2017).

An overly acidic lifestyle through eating processed and other non-real foods has meant that dark, green, leafy vegetables have come into their own for enhanced bone health and muscle retention: they are an excellent source of calcium, vitamin D and other nutrients that can mitigate against the debilitating disease of osteoporosis, a scourge of the Western world (Weaver, 2013: 25). Also, veggies are fibre and fibre makes for excellent gut health according to Dr Libby Weaver (2016a). Weaver explains that the fibre binds to toxic waste products allowing for efficient elimination (aka healthy pooing).

So, strike up a friendship with your greengrocer for a healthier life into your golden years.

3. Washing fruit and vegetables before consumption

Unless they're homegrown or organically grown (and you're not using pesticides), it's a very good idea to wash your fruits and vegetables in a water/vinegar solution before eating them. The reason? You've probably noticed the gleam on the apples, the shine on the oranges or the vibrant and 'healthy' glow of the greens in the supermarket. This is generally achieved during the growing and harvesting phases through the use of pesticides, and it comes at a price: pesticide residue remains on the surface of the fruit and vegetables and cannot easily be removed through water rinsing alone. While pesticides have been tested before human consumption of the produce, with long-term consumption of such produce it's best to eliminate any residue. Pesticides are fat-soluble and so water alone is not sufficient. Weaver (2013: 30) recommends that you fill your sink with water (three parts water, one part vinegar) to soak your produce, then rinse and pat dry before storing or consuming. The vinegar provides that extra element of pesticide elimination, and you can munch your way through your healthy fruits and veggies with a great deal more confidence in their health benefits.

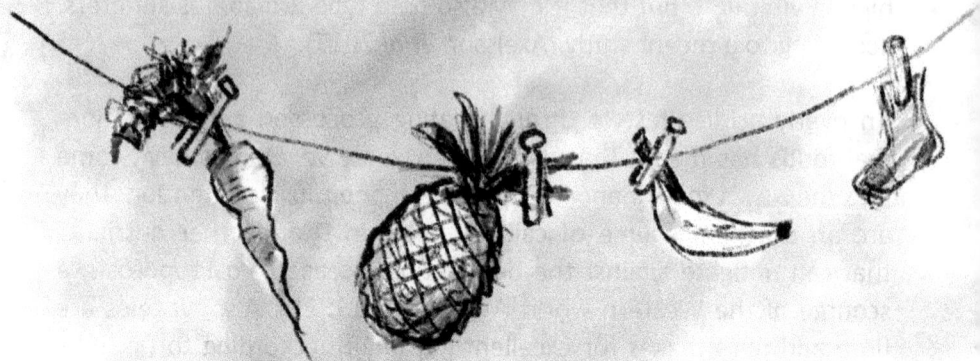

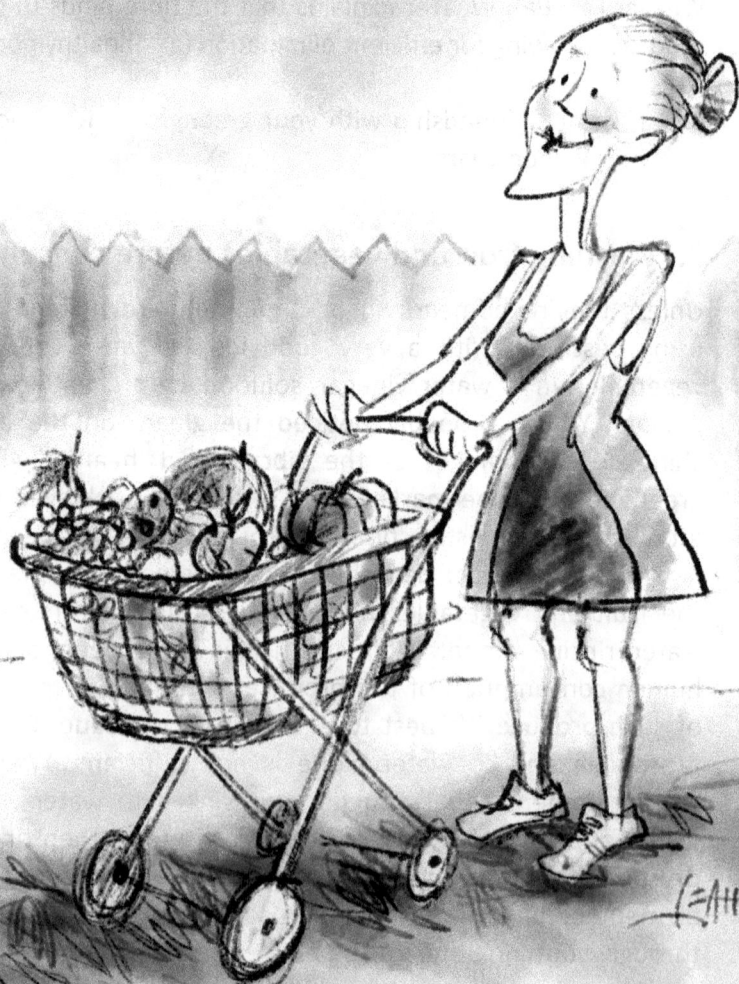

4. Quit the world's most popular drug: sugar

I'm going to suggest, right up front, that you avoid sugar as you would... [insert your own worst nightmare here]. Mine is anything marked with a skull and crossbones symbol. I make no apologies for this dire comparison. However, my hope is not to frighten you but, unapologetically, to warn you of the consequences of prolonged sugar consumption. To borrow and render a distorted version of Dylan Thomas' poem: *Do not go gentle into that good night, but rage against the serious consequences of refined sugars.*

I was first alerted to the poisonous nature of sugar when I read David Gillespie's book *Sweet Poison,* a very readable and credible text that linked sugar to our soaring obesity levels and to some of the chronic diseases that have flourished in the twentieth and twenty-first centuries. If you've ever watched episodes on television of the animated sitcom, *The Simpsons,* you'll appreciate the addictive nature of sugar when Homer downs a box of doughnuts, greedily hunting down the euphoria the sugar treat delivers.

Eminent paediatric endocrinologist Dr Robert Lustig (2016) and urology professor Dr David Samadi (2017) both argue that sugar affects the brain in much the same way as heroin and cocaine. When consuming excessive levels of sugar (as with addictive drugs), there is a change in the gene expression for opioids. Dopamine, the main chemical in the reward system in our brain, is rocketed into overdrive every time an addictive substance is consumed, causing us to seek this 'high' repeatedly, aka addiction (Webster, 2018).

Sugar is believed to be one of the leading causes of ill-health in our modern times (Yudkin, 1972; Lustig, 2016). In the last 30 years, type 2 diabetes rates have tripled to 347 million people worldwide (Hozer, 2016). One million of those are Australians! There's said to be another 500,000 Australians unreported and undiagnosed, and at least another two million who are pre-diabetic (Diabetes Australia, 2015; Graham, 2017). Basically, our food supply has been sweetened (read: *poisoned*) by the food industry. As I've stressed above, sugar is highly addictive, and it is present in almost 80% of the foods on

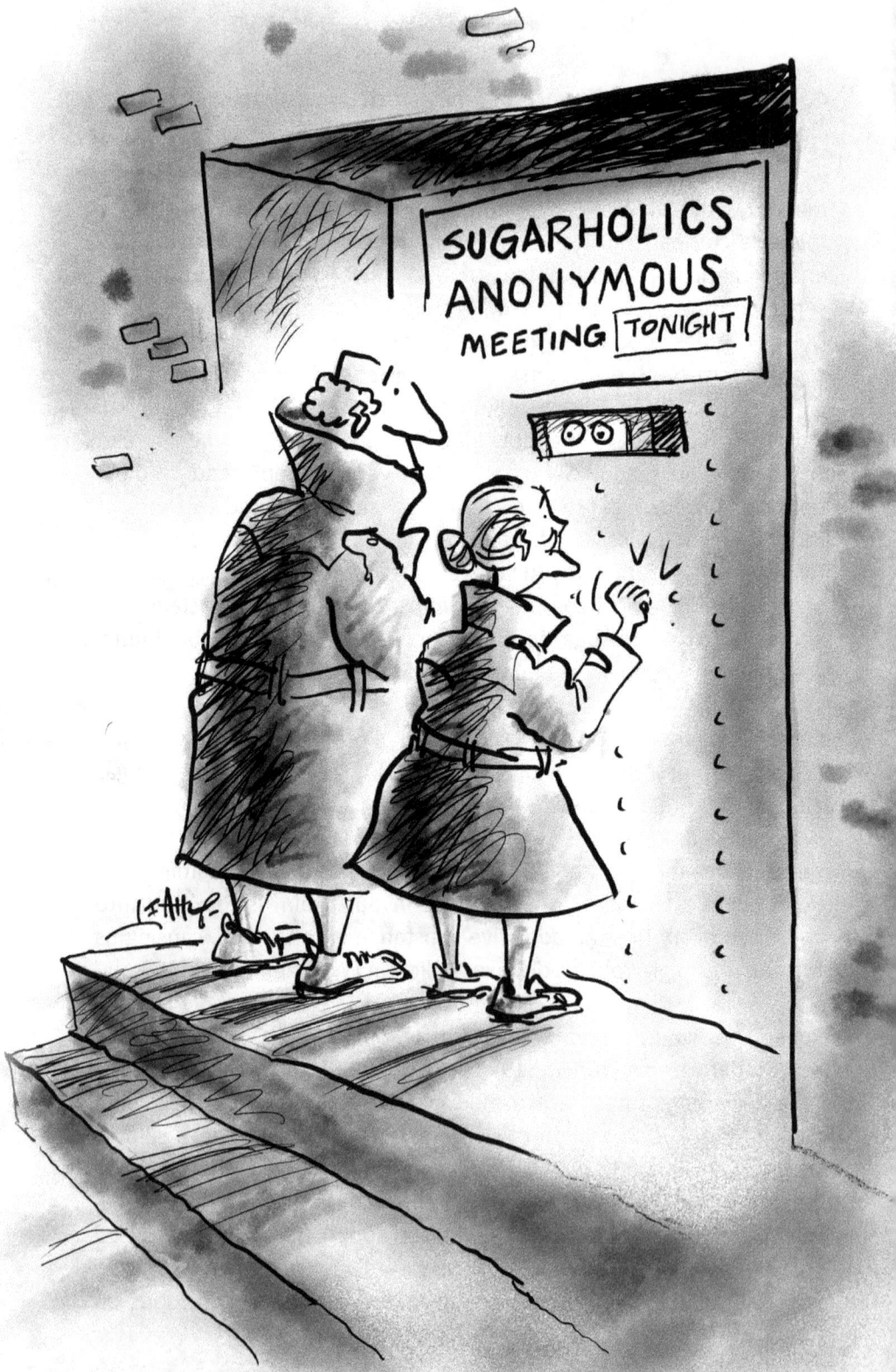

supermarket shelves. They're called processed foods. Your kitchen staples such as breads, tomato sauce, salad dressings, and cereals are often laden with sugar. Just recently I learned that one of my favoured Indian restaurants adds sugar to their mild curries to tame the spiciness. And here I was thinking they had vats of mild, medium and hot sitting on the grill for all tastes! The waitress advised me to order medium if I wanted to avoid added sugar.

There are currently 56 different names that the food industry has ascribed to sugar, perhaps as a way of disguising the culprit of so many of our current health challenges. Look for these sugar-disguised names when checking out the labels on food. They include: *agave nectar, Barbados sugar, barley malt, beet sugar, blackstrap molasses, brown rice syrup, brown sugar, buttered syrup, cane juice crystals, cane sugar, caramel, carob syrup, castor sugar, confectioner's sugar, corn syrup, corn syrup solids, crystalline fructose, date sugar, Demerara sugar, dextran, dextrose, diastatic malt, diatase, ethyl maltol, evaporated cane juice, Florida Crystals, fructose, fruit juice, fruit juice concentrate, galactose, glucose, glucose solids, golden sugar, golden syrup, grape sugar, high-fructose corn syrup, honey, icing sugar, invert sugar, lactose, malt syrup, maltose, maple syrup, molasses, muscovado sugar, organic raw sugar, panocha, raw sugar, refiner's syrup, rice syrup, sorghum syrup, sucrose, sugar, treacle, turbinado sugar and yellow sugar* (Lustig, 2013; Cityline, 2017).

As Lustig would say, we've all been 'frucked' by Big Sugar. He is a powerful lobbyist for the case against sugar consumption and its disguises in our foods. I'm a strong advocate for what he's got to say. The battle that he faces (and it's *our* battle as well) is akin to the one that Jeffrey Wigand faced against the tobacco industry in the 1990s. The Hollywood film *The Insider* (1999), starring Al Pacino and Russell Crowe, brought the corrupt and life-threatening underbelly of the tobacco industry into sharp and painful focus. However, whereas sectors of the cigarette-smoking public (and passive-smoking public) are negatively impacted by tobacco, sugar consumption has an almost blanket consumption across the population, often hidden in the many processed foods that shroud the supermarket shelves.

According to 2017 statistics, Australia is the fifth most overweight and obese OECD country: we have 11 million adults and one million children considered overweight or obese! That's two in every three Aussies with a very unhealthy body mass index (BMI) (Carrano, 2017). Obesity levels in Australia have risen from 19% of adults in 1995 to 28% in 2014–15. I believe sugar is the source of much of this problem. Lustig has been arguing for years that sugar is a poison that is wreaking havoc on our health in a range of sinister forms: obesity, heart disease, cancer! But do not despair: the effects of sugar consumption on your health can be reversed very easily if you act before disease sets in. Markedly reducing sugar intake has been shown to have immediate and positive results on overall health. A study on 43 African-American and Latino children who were diagnosed with metabolic syndrome (obesity) saw dramatic weight loss and a reduction in blood pressure and LDL (bad) cholesterol levels in just 10 days. They effectively reduced their risk of type 2 diabetes (Lustig *et al*, 2016).

Another important point I want to reiterate from Lustig's philosophy is that *not all calories are created equal*. Eating 100 calories of sugar and 100 calories of, say, broccoli, is not the same. Your body processes those two foods in very different ways; burning off that sugar requires much more energy than burning off your greens. But the big food companies want you to believe the lie: that's why they promote low-calorie food items with the suggestion that they're better for you. Wrong! While sugar is not fat, it converts to fat in your body, especially if your liver is overloaded with sugar.

I've probably rattled on a little with this topic, but it's because I'm so passionate about getting across the message about the pervasiveness of sugar in our culture and the danger of sugar consumption to our health. It's now an issue that the Australian Medical Association (AMA) is finally taking seriously. In January 2018, the then-AMA President, Dr Michael Gannon, publicly acknowledged the widespread damage being caused by an overconsumption of sugar in this country. While Gannon stopped short of demonising sugar altogether, stating that "consumption is not a problem in and of itself", he recognised that it is a "significant contributor to the obesity epidemic we are facing [in Australia]" (Hunter, 2018). What the AMA proposes is banning advertising of junk food, taxing sweetened drinks and removing from medical facilities vending machines containing unhealthy food products. Finally, someone with the profile and power in this country to make a change has spoken up.

If you're finding it difficult to navigate the food world and distinguish what's sugar and what's not, then you'll be pleased to know about some emerging technology that allows you to track the food you put in your mouth. It's called 'Tooth Fitbits' and it's a food tracker that is mounted on your tooth and is easily removable, allowing you to track in real time the amount of sugar, salt and alcohol you're consuming. The data is then sent straight to your mobile phone (Gollayan, 2018).

To conclude this rant, let me just say that *the brief pleasure that sugar brings is not worth its long-term health-damaging effects.* If you want to read an interesting article about the benefits of eliminating sugar, you can't go past Alanna Ketler's article (Ketler, 2016). Please see my *Green juicing* section for a good detox once you make the decision to cut down sugar or cut it out from your healthy eating plan. Enough said!

5. Eating the rainbow

Sounds lovely, doesn't it! You don't need to go searching for that elusive rainbow after a storm or sun shower, or emulate Dorothy seeking her magic mile 'somewhere over the rainbow'. Your rainbow is all the colourful fruits and vegetables that nature has provided, along with nuts, seeds and extra-virgin olive oil. It also consists of fish two to three times a week and occasionally, red meat. Fish and other seafood, like red meat, contain plenty of protein to build muscle as well as healthy fats to decrease your risk of heart disease and stroke (McKay, 2017). Another name for the rainbow diet is a Mediterranean diet – full of colour and vitality. Phytochemicals are the natural chemicals that give fruit and vegetables their colours, and these offer a diverse range of nutrients and health benefits. Five serves of vegetables and two of fruit is the recommended portions for us to eat each day (AMA, *Nutrition*, 2018).

So, eating one of each of the six main colours of fruit and veg daily helps you meet your necessary nutrient requirements. The best part about this diet is that it is known to ward off chronic illness and depression: those who eat the rainbow are believed to be happier and to live longer (Better Health Channel, 2016). And there's the cost savings as well. A recent Deakin University study suggests an annual saving of around AUD2,591 when taking into account reduced grocery bills, fewer health professional visits and thus less travel time, and less time off work (Van den Berg, 2018). Now, there's your pot of gold! Below, I've tabled the colours, their nutritional benefits and the various vegetable and fruit sources to make it easier for you to colour your world for a healthier you.

Colour	Nutrients/Elements	Sources/Benefits
Red	Antioxidants	Tomatoes, red berries such as strawberries & raspberries, pomegranates: protect cells from damage
Orange	Carotenoids— alpha-carotene & betacarotene (Vitamin A) & beta-cryptoxanthin, an antioxidant	Pumpkin, sweet potato, carrots: protect against cellular damage, aging and some chronic diseases
Yellow	Antioxidants— Betacarotene & beta-cryptoxanthin	Grapefruit, lemon, pineapple, sweet corn, button squash, yellow capsicum: reduce risk of developing inflammatory diseases such as rheumatoid arthritis

Green	Fibre, vitamins, minerals	Spinach, broccoli, peas, kale: contain lutein and zeaxanthin for age-related eye disease. Broccoli, cabbage, Brussels sprouts, kale, pak choi: protection against certain cancers & blood vessel damage
Blue/Purple	Antioxidants— Anthocyanins	Beetroot, radishes, purple cabbage, carrots, beans, blueberries: anthocyanins protect against cell damage & reduce risk of cancer, stroke & heart disease
White/Brown	Anthoxanthins	Dates, mushrooms, fennel, garlic, lychees: reduce risk of cardiovascular disease & arthritis. Banana and parsnip: potassium for heart & muscle function. Cauliflower, turnip, cabbage: cancer fighter, strengthening bone tissue & maintaining healthy blood vessels

Source: Better Health Channel (2016)

6. Vegetable juicing

I discovered green juicing many years ago but didn't take any action on it, not then recognising and appreciating the amazing health benefits of vegetable juicing until more recently. Several years ago I read a book that advocated green juicing as a powerful and effective way to alkalise your body, reduce weight and boost the necessary nutrients in your daily diet to provide the foundation for a healthy body. Since then, I've been to a health coach who said exactly the same thing as I'd read years earlier, especially about how important green juicing is to attain and maintain a healthy pH by reducing inflammation in the body which would otherwise lead to disease.

You'll note I emphasise *vegetable* juicing as opposed to juicing fruits. Fruits become pure fructose once juiced which can lead to insulin resistance and would otherwise, I believe, neutralise the value of your green vegetable juicing. So, for the past two years or so I've been vegetable juicing and I love it. I purchased my centrifugal juicer, set it up on the kitchen bench as a permanent fixture and followed my health coach's recipe for cleansing and nourishing. You'll get all the nutrients you need in a glass of vegetable juice; you'll be able to consume way more vegetables and in a greater variety than you could possibly put on your plate; it'll build your immune system, increase your energy levels and support brain function. All that in a glass of vegetable juice!

Since purchasing my juicer, I've done further research into alternatives: cold-press juicers. The distinction between a cold-press and centrifugal juice extractor is that a centrifugal extractor utilises a fast-spinning metal blade that destroys some of the enzymes. Consequently, heat is generated that oxidises the nutrients, rendering a less nutritious juice. A cold-press juicer, on the other hand, crushes the vegetable matter and gives a higher juice yield, generating much less heat so the nutrients stay intact. Of course, cost is the big factor between centrifugal and cold-press juicers, the latter being on the higher end. Nevertheless, irrespective of which juicer you choose or can afford, juicing is an important inclusion in any healthy eating plan.

I offer two simple juice recipes below to get you started. One has a fruit option, but the other is pure vegetable juice, which is my preference:

Dr Jocker's Beginners Green Juice
3–4 celery stalks
1–2 cucumbers (peeled)
Parsley (go easy on this strong flavoured green)
½ lemon (the citric acid lowers the glycaemic impact of the inflammatory component of the fructose in the juice)
½ knob ginger
1 green apple (optional)

Dr Thomas Bige's Vegetable Juice
Carrots (purple if you can get them)
Cucumber (peeled)
Beetroot
Cabbage (red, preferably)
Silverbeet
Kale
Celery
Ginger

7. The colour purple

Purple plant foods are the secret elixir to a long life and they are worthy of being singled out. In particular, I'd like to discuss the purple sweet potato. Regular consumption of the purple vegetable is said to deliver a long and disease-free life. Just ask the Okinawan people in Japan. The BBC1 documentary, *How to Stay Young,* explained that Okinawa boasts the largest number of centenarians in the world (Binding, 2016). In fact, Japan has a record 67,824 centenarians at time of writing (Edmistone, 2017). One of their major vegetable staples is the humble purple sweet potato. They even have purple sweet potato ice-cream!

Internationally recognised expert in healthy aging, Professor Craig Wilcox, undertook in 2001 the 'Okinawan Centenarian Study' and his findings suggest that purple sweet potatoes are the "powerhouses of nutrition". Along with longevity, the Okinawan elders have a very low incidence of chronic aging diseases such as Alzheimer's, cardiovascular disease and cancer. It is also believed that other fruits and vegetables distinguished by their deep blue and purple colouring are excellent sources of antioxidants, translating into a healthier life: blackberries, blueberries, blackcurrants, purple carrots, purple cabbage, and so on. And while we're discussing the Okinawan people, you might like to know that they follow an interesting philosophy which might also be linked to their longevity. It's called *hara hachi bu* (eight parts out of ten) and it governs their meals, meaning they stop eating when they're 80% full (Glassman,

2014). One 100-year-old Okinawan local summed up the secret to his youthful vigour: "Food is medicine," he declared. Now that's a message that's easy to swallow.

8. Drinking water

Drinking water is so vital to optimum health that you'd think drinking it would be a straightforward process. And it is – for the most part! There are a number of points of view about how much you should drink, how you should drink it, what temperature to drink it at, the benefits and the drawbacks. Since I don't think it's fair that I should be alone at this watershed moment, I'm going to share these simple and helpful ideas with you.

According to Dr Libby Weaver (2016: 47–48), our bodies are predominantly made up of water. Our lungs are 90% water, the brain is 76% water and our bones contain 25% water. Water is life to our bodies and imperative for good health. While there is some conflict over how much water we should drink each day, the current science suggests that we need 33 millilitres (ml) for each kg of body weight. So a 75-kg individual requires 2,475 ml, or roughly 2½ L per day.

It's been argued that in order to give your body a good detoxification, you should drink at least a couple of glasses of water before eating breakfast. Too often, we rely on exercise to eliminate toxins – generally through our skin! What a tough call to make on our skin, the largest organ in our body! Rather, by drinking water in the morning you're flushing your kidneys and giving your colon a good cleanse, which in turn more easily allows your body to eliminate waste through the bowel and urethra (Wolfe, 2016).

According to Ayurvedic tradition, you should sit rather than stand to drink water, but this is a contentious issue, with other traditions professing the opposite. I encourage you to research this yourself, but I believe the most important message is simply to be drinking water, whether it's in the seated or standing position. Drink slowly, tepid water not cold, drink when thirsty, sip small amounts of water while eating, but avoid drinking water just after eating as it diminishes the energy of our digestive system to process the food – also, the food will remain longer in our systems, causing it to rot and leading to gas and acidity problems (CureJoy Editorial, 2016).

Drink a glass of warm water before a shower to lower blood pressure. The warmth of the water that you drink combined with the warmth of the water in the hot bath or shower serves to dilate your blood vessels, causing your blood pressure to drop. The water that you drink also dilutes your body's sodium levels, which further decreases blood pressure. So a glass of water before a hot bath or shower really can help your health! (To Lower Blood Pressure, 2012). Of course, if you have a heart condition or blood pressure issues, then it's best to check in with your doctor first (Steber, 2018).

If you drink alcohol, it amps up dehydration, so it's a good idea to alternate between a glass of alcohol and a glass of water to be sure to stay hydrated (Weaver, 2016: 60).

Drink filtered water if possible. A good filtration system will bring the water to a more alkaline state between eight and nine. As mentioned elsewhere in this book, an acidic state of the body is a breeding ground for disease. My benchtop filter system removes contaminants such as heavy metals, pesticides and chlorine, and includes essential minerals: magnesium, potassium, calcium, manganese, and sodium.

Make it warm water! I know I've mentioned warm water just before a shower, but choosing to drink warm rather than cold water on every occasion is best. (I know, you're thinking, arghhh, I can't drink warm water especially in a hot climate.) But your mission, should you choose to accept it, will lead to better blood circulation, flushing out of toxins (including those pesky fat deposits), enhanced circulation, and greater muscle relaxation, which all improve blood flow. And the great thing is, neither you nor this message will self-destruct within 30 seconds of reading!

9. Drinking green tea

Many years ago, I read the book *Eat Right for your Blood Type* by Dr Peter D'Adamo. I'm an O negative blood type. Among his many other recommendations, Dr D'Adamo suggested that with this blood type, black tea or coffee was taboo, but that green and other herbal teas were much more therapeutic. So I ditched the black tea and coffee and have been drinking green tea ever since. At the time, I didn't know about the amazing health benefits derived from drinking green tea. It's loaded with polyphenols like flavonoids and catechins: these operate as powerful antioxidants. Antioxidants cleanse the body of toxins, which cause disease in the body. Disease manifests as cancers and other breakdowns in the body. Other amazing benefits include enhanced brain function through its small amounts of caffeine and the amino acid L-theanine. It also boosts your metabolic rate for fat burning and weight loss (Gunnars, 2017).

One of the best green teas on the market is said to be matcha. It's a traditional ceremonial tea from Japan and is more nutrient dense than regular green tea (Sass, 2015). So, when you're at the supermarket next time, pick up a pack of green tea, or better still, get the green loose leaf tea or matcha if you can find it. And speaking of the kettle, there's one other important consideration when making your green tea: don't allow the water to boil, or if you do, let it cool a little before pouring it onto the tea. The tea tastes much better, preventing that bitterness sometimes associated with green tea. There are even temperature-controlled kettles that you adjust for your preferences, so you'll get the perfect temperature for whatever tea you're brewing. Just a note of encouragement to use loose leaf tea rather than the teabag variety. I've recently learned that many teabag brands use small amounts of plastic known as polypropylene to seal the teabags and retain their shape in boiling water (Spinks, 2018). As I see it, there are two problems with this. The first is that toxic chemicals known as phthalates are released when heat meets plastic, which messes with your hormones. Secondly, there is the environmental factor when considering the millions of teabags that make their way into landfills or compost bins – plastic does not break down like organic materials. Reassuringly, some manufacturers are looking for non-plastic alternatives. So, with all this in mind, why don't you pop the kettle on? You'll be glad you did, and you might end up becoming a green tea fan. Your body and your overall health will thank you. And if you don't believe me, perhaps you'll trust the wisdom of third-oldest Australian 110-year-old Phyllis Lee (as at 3 November 2017), who attributes her good health and longevity to "drinking...lots of cups of tea" (Edmistone, 2017). Now, where's that kettle. I'll be mother...

10. All you can beet: beetroot

Beetroot gets a special mention because of its amazing health and wellbeing-enhancing qualities. Beetroot's right up there with the best of them. I'm talking about fresh, raw beetroot with stems, not beetroot in a can. My understanding is that most canned beetroots are loaded with sugar, which neutralises the healthy benefits of this vegetable. Unlike many of my readers, perhaps, I'm a relative latecomer to the raw and real beetroot phenomenon, having only recognised its worth when I started juicing. Nevertheless, it's an ancient root vegetable, hailed by the father of medicine, Hippocrates, for its wound-healing properties. It was also lauded in the Middle Ages as a treatment for digestive and blood disorders, and now it is embraced in contemporary Aussie culture at barbeques and banquets for its goodness and flavour (McGrath, 2017). More recently, beetroot has been hailed as a meaningful performance enhancer among athletes; the nitrate in beetroot juice is said to improve "the efficiency of processes that occur in the mitochondria, which are the cell's energy factory" (Peeling, 2016). In other words, beetroot can give an explosive edge to an athlete. According to Associate Professor Peter Peeling of the University of Western Australia, beetroot consumption in field-based tests gave the participants a 1.7% performance enhancement. Doesn't seem like much, does it, until you consider the 2012 Olympic Games kayaking races cited by Peeling, with the margin between gold and silver medallists in the men's K1-1000m and the women's K1-500m races at 0.3% and 1.0% respectively. For the supreme athletes among you, you can't 'beet' that! But for the rest of us mere mortals, there's still a lot to be up-beet about when it comes to this red vegetable for enhancing our health.

According to dietitian Rebecca Flavel (McGrath, 2017), beetroot's packed full of vitamins (C and B6, folate, manganese, betaine, and potassium), minerals, antioxidants, and fibre. It also has powerful antioxidant, detoxification and anti-inflammatory qualities, and as mentioned with our athletes earlier, the nitrates help our muscles use oxygen more efficiently.

In juicing terms, beetroot juice aids our liver in eliminating damaging toxins while stimulating the liver cells. And for the beauty-conscious among us, it offers some protection against the aging process by neutralising free radicals, and lycopene helps keep the skin supple. It really is a case of 'you are what you beet'! And just when you thought it's appropriate to throw away the leafy greens attached to the beetroot, don't! They're packed with vitamins and minerals far in excess of the beetroot itself. Why don't you toss them into your next salad to give a boost to your iron intake? One note of caution here though: as beetroot leaves contain high levels of oxalates, for those who have kidney stones please limit your intake, so you don't build up this organic acid in the urine (National Kidney Foundation, 2017). For those who don't need to avoid this, there's just one more benefit I'd like to mention in association with this humble but valuable root. The nitrates mentioned earlier are said to increase blood flow and sex drive. Beetroot, you see, contains the mineral boron which the ancient Romans used as an early form of Viagra to boost their libido. Why don't you *beet* a path to your greengrocer today and ask for the beet, and nothing but the beet?

11. Lemon juice and apple cider vinegar

This was one of the first health tips I was introduced to when I started seriously looking at my health and needing to do some things differently. Lemon juice, a rich source of vitamin C, and apple cider vinegar, although acidic in nature, have an alkalising effect on the body and a range of medicinal benefits. Both contain powerful antibacterial and antiviral properties for boosting the immune system. They're also brilliant digestive and detoxifying agents, helping to clean the liver. For excellent gut health, I drink either a teaspoon of apple cider vinegar with water, or the juice of half a lemon in warm water first thing in the morning about half an hour before eating. The lemon juice wakes up the liver so it flushes out toxins, stimulates digestion, supports weight loss, and soothes an upset tummy. One tip: if you're using both cold and hot water to mix, then put the cold water in first then the hot, otherwise you will kill the valuable enzymes in the lemon juice. A diluted mix of apple cider vinegar and water can also mildly reduce bacteria colonies such as *Staphylococcus aureus* and *Pseudomonas aeruginosa* that are implicated in inflammatory conditions like leaky gut syndrome.

Also, don't sip, just drink it down, as dentists warn that the acid from lemons or vinegar could damage tooth enamel. Simply rinsing your mouth with water after drinking will remove any acid from the enamel. Or better still, why not drink the lemon juice or apple cider vinegar through a reusable metal straw, being kind to our environment while protecting our teeth at the same time. Both the lemon juice and apple cider vinegar are brilliant at supporting a more alkaline pH. Either one is a great way to kick-start your system each day (Cole, 2017).

12. pH balance

Having a pH in your blood of 80/20 alkaline/acidic is essential for overall optimum health. pH stands for 'power of hydrogen' – a measure of the hydrogen ion concentration in the body. An imbalance of alkaline/acidity in the body allows unhealthy organisms to thrive, destroys tissues and organs and compromises the immune system. In their publication *The pH Miracle* (2002), Dr Robert O Young and Shelley Young argue that this 80/20 ideal translates into a typical alkaline diet consisting of 80% alkaline foods and 20% acidic foods. An ideal pH is slightly alkaline, between 7.30–7.45. Eating raw fruit and vegetables that are more alkaline will help you achieve this balance. Raw is a better option when compared with their cooked cousins: if you prefer cooked then try to stir-fry or short-steam your vegetables. Tea, coffee and highly processed foods all contribute to an acidic state. You can help alkalise your body by adding natural mineral salts to your food, such as Himalayan or Celtic salts. A pinch of sodium bicarbonate in a glass of water will alkalise the water (and you). And one of my favourites mentioned earlier is freshly squeezed lemon juice in a glass of water. This not only helps attain an alkaline state but is also great for digestion.

A more acidic body is exacerbated by emotional triggers such as stress, so addressing your stress rather than ignoring or suppressing it is a marvellous way to a more balanced pH. Furthermore, mixing high protein foods with carbohydrates, starches or sugars in the same meal also increases an acidic state.

You can test your pH levels by simply purchasing pH test strip papers from an online pharmacy or local pharmacy and conducting either a saliva or urine test. For a saliva test, you simply discharge some saliva into a plastic spoon, place the pH strip into the saliva and then compare the colour of your immersed pH strip with the colour chart provided with your pH papers. Be sure not to have eaten or drunk anything within half an hour of testing, and it's a good idea to be consistent with your timing of the test, such as in the mornings when you wake. This way you can chart the trend of your pH.

I've included a link to a pH chart (PRD Enterprises, 2013) in the *Reference List* with a list of typical foods and liquids and their level of alkalinity or acidity. Keep it handy, perhaps on the fridge in the kitchen, for easy checking. At time of writing, the charts were available online for AUD17.95.

13. Don't miss it: breakfast

You've more than likely heard the adage that breakfast is the most important meal of the day. From my own experience, I have to agree. It's an important cultural practice that dates back to the Middle Ages. To adapt what 1960's nutritionist Adelle Davis famously announced, it's important we eat breakfast like a king or queen, lunch like a prince or princess and eat dinner like a pauper (Sifferlin, 2016). While we all need to aim to fuel our tanks with *at least* 25% of our daily energy intake first up in the morning, there are a good many of us (around 25%) who don't eat breakfast at all, and for adolescents in North America it's as high as 36% skipping this important meal (Spencer, 2017; Seiga-Riz *et al,* 1998). The Australian Bureau of Statistics (ABS) revealed that here in Australia, one in seven children either skips breakfast or goes to school hungry (O'Neil *et al*, 2014). About three years ago in a class I was teaching, I discovered this to be true. I ran an informal survey of my 12 and 13-year-old students, following a nutritional talk by the school counsellor. I asked the students to put up their hands if they hadn't eaten breakfast that morning. About one-third of the students in a class of 24 raised their hands. It was a disturbing discovery.

What is the reasoning behind breakfast's privileged role by they-who-know-best? A healthy breakfast sets you up for the day, promotes weight maintenance and weight loss and regulates blood glucose levels and your metabolism. Conversely, for those who skip breakfast, the American Heart Association warns that there's the risk of obesity, heart disease and diabetes (Spencer, 2017). Moreover, the failure to eat a well-balanced and nutritional breakfast is said to impede cognitive performance. Academically, that's worrying. By eating a nutritional breakfast, you'll improve your alertness, concentration, mental acuity, mood, and memory (O'Neil, 2014). Whether you're studying, working or just trying to navigate your way around the world, breakfast is a meal you shouldn't miss. As the name suggests, you're *breaking the fast* after resting overnight for around eight hours, which is an extended time without eating.

Food is energy and your get-up-and-go will have got-up-and-gone if you don't fuel your body for the day ahead. My breakfast consists of eggs and vegetables such as mushrooms, tomatoes, spinach, and avocado with a side of gluten-free toast occasionally if I'm extra-hungry after a swim. The Dietitians Association of Australia (2018) recommends the following range of brekky ideas: whole grain cereal with milk, yoghurt, fresh fruit, and a sprinkle of nuts; fresh fruit smoothie with yoghurt and milk; toasted sourdough with cheese, baked beans and avocado; untoasted muesli or rolled oats; poached eggs on wholegrain toast with tomato, spinach and mushrooms. If your focus is on weight loss, then you'll be keen to know that eating a nutritious breakfast reduces your blood sugar levels, preventing binge eating later in the day that would otherwise lead to weight gain.

A five-year American study of 12,000 individuals evaluated breakfast consumption, overall energy intake and BMI with a recommendation in favour of breakfast consumption because it was associated with improved diet quality, diet energy density and body weight (Kant et al, 2008). The findings of another five-year study of 2,200 adolescents that looked at the association between breakfast frequency and healthy weight resulted in a recommendation to support adolescents in eating breakfast regularly (Timlin et al, 2008; Seiga-Riz et al, 1998).

A cautionary note regarding breakfast cereals. Queensland cancer surgeon, Dr Andrew Renaut, has witnessed the adverse effects of poor diet on his patients. He uses the term 'cereal killer' to describe many breakfast cereals and says that these and other processed foods are packed full of sugar, which has an undeniable link between obesity and an increase in some cancers, heart attacks, stroke, diabetes, and Alzheimer's disease (Passmore, 2018).

By now, you're probably saying that all this information is well and good, but I haven't got the time, or I don't feel hungry in the mornings. I get it! But a little planning and some creative ideas to entice the tastebuds might be all the inspiration you need. Getting up just 10 minutes earlier than usual to have a breakfast such as fruit, or vegetables from the previous evening, are ways around the problem. Making an on-the-go breakfast of thick oatmeal, topping it with nuts and/or fruit and placing it in a travel mug that will fit in your car's console or travel well on public transport can save you the eating time at home. If it's an omelette you're thinking of, cutting up and preparing your omelette vegetables the night before and having all your cutlery and utensils set up in the kitchen ready to go will make breakfast more seamless. You could also shop for the week, planning your breakfast meals and factoring in nutrition and ease (Produce for Better Health Foundation, 2018). Many restaurants and cafés have all-day breakfast menus now to satisfy the 'breakfastarians' among us. As food critic and columnist A A Gill put it, "Breakfast is everything. The beginning, the first thing. It is the mouthful that is the commitment to a new day, a continuing life" (Gerrard, 2016).

14. Vitamin C: the wonder vitamin

I recently watched the documentary *Food Matters* (2008) in which doctors, naturopaths, nutritionists, and journalists expressed concerns about the lack of nutrition in our current diets, despite the abundance of food we have access to. What figures significantly in the film is the health benefits of vitamin C (aka ascorbic acid). As our bodies are incapable of generating vitamin C naturally, we rely on receiving it through our foods. Fruits and vegetables such as citrus fruits and leafy green vegetables are the obvious sources. It's best to eat these vegetables raw where possible, or with minimal cooking to preserve the benefits of the vitamin C. However, as the trace elements are not always available in the soils that our food is grown in, or the vitamins and minerals are depleted due to pesticides, a 1000 mg vitamin C tablet each day may be the way to supplement your vitamin C fix. I would encourage you not to replace fresh fruit and vegetables with a pill, but rather to supplement where needed.

So what do these health professionals claim are the health benefits of vitamin C? It aids in the prevention and treatment of scurvy (don't scoff, scurvy is still a problem for Australian health today), the common cold, building your immune system, controlling asthma symptoms, addressing and reducing lead toxicity, treating cataracts, stroke and cancer, and for maintaining the skin's elasticity. The medical specialists in *Food Matters* explain that high doses of vitamin C are required to address some of these ailments and diseases, but for general wellbeing and staving off illnesses, ascorbic acid may well be the perfect pill (or a fruit and veggie source) for you.

15. Quinoa, the superfood

Pronounced *keen-wah*, it has been around for thousands of years and was the staple diet of the ancient Incas and their descendants. This superfood is said to be packed with nutrition. In recognition of this nutrient-rich content, the UN even named 2013 'International Quinoa Year'! It's an excellent source of calcium, magnesium and manganese, packed with several B vitamins, vitamin E and dietary fibre. Quinoa is also a complete protein (containing all nine essential amino acids) that's wheat-free – great news for those with coeliac disease and the gluten-intolerant among us. While looking like a grain, it's actually a seed from the same family as beets, spinach and chard. Quinoa has anti-inflammatory phytonutrients that work to ward off disease. This little food gem has traces of omega-3 fatty acids, essential for the body's function. It's a versatile food that once cooked, can be sprinkled on salads or used in place of couscous or rice. When preparing quinoa, it's preferable to rinse it in a sieve before boiling as the compound that coats the seeds, saponins, will create a foam that has a somewhat bitter taste. There is one downside to quinoa consumption. It is not a health concern but an ethical issue. With such global demand for quinoa, the local Andean population has markedly reduced their diversity of crops in favour of dedicated quinoa fields (Lewin, 2017). I'll leave it to you to determine whether the health benefits outweigh the ethical considerations, especially if your quinoa is sourced from the Andes.

16. Consume extra-virgin olive oil

Four tablespoons of extra-virgin olive oil daily is recommended by Dr Aseem Malhotra, a leading British cardiologist. With some medical professionals now acknowledging that sugar, not fat, makes people fat, Dr Malhotra suggests that the best heart medication is taking a few tablespoons of extra-virgin olive oil daily, a handful of nuts and lots of veggies, and eliminating sugar (my pet aversion).

In the documentary *The Big Fat Fix* (O'Neill, Donal & Malhotra, 2016), Dr Malhotra demonstrates how the consumption of olive oil works to erode the plaque that builds up in our arteries due to a poor diet. Moreover, olive oil contains about 75% of its fat in the form of oleic acid (a monounsaturated, omega-9 fatty acid). There are many benefits to oleic acid that include proper balance of total cholesterol, LDL cholesterol and HDL cholesterol in the body. And there's more good news: the Greeks consume around 20 litres of the stuff each year, compared with Australians with just two litres per year. Their love of olive oil has meant that the Greeks have lower heart disease and obesity. There could be a correlation here between olive oil consumption and better health, don't you think?

This good oil also boosts circulation to all areas of your body. That's said to be a positive pre-condition for an enhanced sex life, among other benefits! And for those who want to retain a glowing skin, olive oil both internally and externally is a must (Jenkins, 2017). Purchasing first-press olive oil is best because the oil retains the delicate flavours and aromas that second and subsequent pressings lack. Often, you will find that the virgin olive oil you purchase from the supermarket has had several pressings before it gets to you.

If you need any convincing about the merits of olive oil and its correlation with a healthy lifespan, look no further than Frenchwoman Jeanne Calment who lived to be 122 years of age. She was said to be the oldest living person until her death in 1997. Jeanne used liberal doses of olive oil daily, boasting that she doused her dinner in olive oil and also lathered it on her skin (Booth, 2013). With so many benefits to olive oil, it is obvious that longevity will be the result. So, pour it on your salads, your scrambled eggs or whatever food you like, and lather it on your body for a healthier, longer-living you.

17. A bitter pill worth swallowing

What I'm referring to here is eating bitter foods. This topic is associated with eating raw and real foods. Because we're so conditioned to eating sweet foods, many of our palates have become averse to the bitter foods. You can reverse this by simply reducing (or preferably, eliminating) processed sugars from your diet to help develop your palate for the finer foods in life. These finer, bitter foods include leafy green vegetables, turmeric, ginger, olives, dark chocolate, and the like. They're called 'bitter' simply because of the action they produce when we eat them: increasing saliva and stomach acids and stimulating the digestive system. That's great news for gut health!

The benefits of bitters were known to the ancient Egyptians, and bitter herbs enhanced the sixteenth-century remedies of renowned Swiss physician Paracelsus. Bitter herbs were brewed as a cure-all but especially as an aid to digestion. You may have heard the expression 'a bitter pill'. Well, far from the negative connotations the phrase may evoke, the term refers to the medicinal benefits derived from these bitter substances. Bitter foods stimulate your liver to produce bile, which aids digestion, and the bile works to emulsify fats – a critical element in the digestive process. Bitters are said to increase the production of digestive enzymes for food absorption and to reduce the risk of leaky gut. A leaky gut means that food particles make their way into the intestines and bloodstream, leading to inflammation. When inflammation becomes chronic, it can lead to various diseases (Newcomer, 2017).

Consuming bitter foods curbs sugar cravings, increases absorption of fat-soluble vitamins A, D, E, and K, helps maintain healthy blood sugar levels, eases constipation, and regulates bowel movements (Grossman, 2018). A couple of caveats to consuming bitters need to be mentioned: if you suffer from acid reflux, stomach ulcers or other digestive issues then you might want to consult your doctor before launching into a diet rich in bitter foods. Oh, and remember, all things in balance and moderation because unfriendly side effects could include bloating and gas with overindulgence (Newcomer, 2017). Having said this, what it all boils down to is the un-bitter truth: eating bitter foods means a happy, healthy gut and that leads to a healthier you (Weaver, 2016a).

18. The magic of turmeric

Turmeric or *Curcuma longa* is a bright-yellow powdery spice extensively used as a powerful anti-inflammatory agent in Chinese and Indian medicine. Its benefits are as broad as they are varied. It is said to aid in the treatment of flatulence (who wouldn't want a little less of this), jaundice, menstrual difficulties, bloody urine, haemorrhage, toothache, bruises, chest pain, and colic. The primary agent in turmeric is curcumin, which gives it the bright-yellow colour, but it does so much more than just colour food. Curcumin's potent anti-inflammatory effects are said to be comparable to over-the-counter anti-inflammatory medicines but without the potential toxic side effects. In line with its anti-inflammatory properties, curcumin's anti-cancer activity has been revealed by medical studies. It is said to be effective on a range of biological pathways (Wilken *et al*, 2011). I sprinkle turmeric on all my dishes and even on my breakfast foods and yoghurt. It is best eaten with a source of fat because it's fat-soluble: the active ingredient, curcumin, can only dissolve in fat in order to make its way to the gut where the immune system resides. When I broke my wrist a few years ago, I was told about the beneficial effects of making a poultice using turmeric, which helped to reduce the inflammation and consolidate the excellent work of my orthopaedic surgeon. If you want to learn more about this amazing spice, just Google 'George Mateljan Foundation' and 'turmeric'. The *Reference List* at the end of this book provides further details. Sprinkle on a little turmeric. It's like fairy dust: just as magical, but more powerful.

19. Bone broth: a health and beauty boost

Perhaps you've got recollections of your grandma making you bone broth, especially when you were feeling unwell. You may recall how comforting as well as healing it was. That time-honoured tradition has had a resurgence today and become uber-trendy. NBA champion, Kobe Bryant, and Australian actress and former supermodel, Elle MacPherson, both attest to the magic of bone broth that goes way beyond a remedy for coughs and colds (Anthony, 2017). The tradition

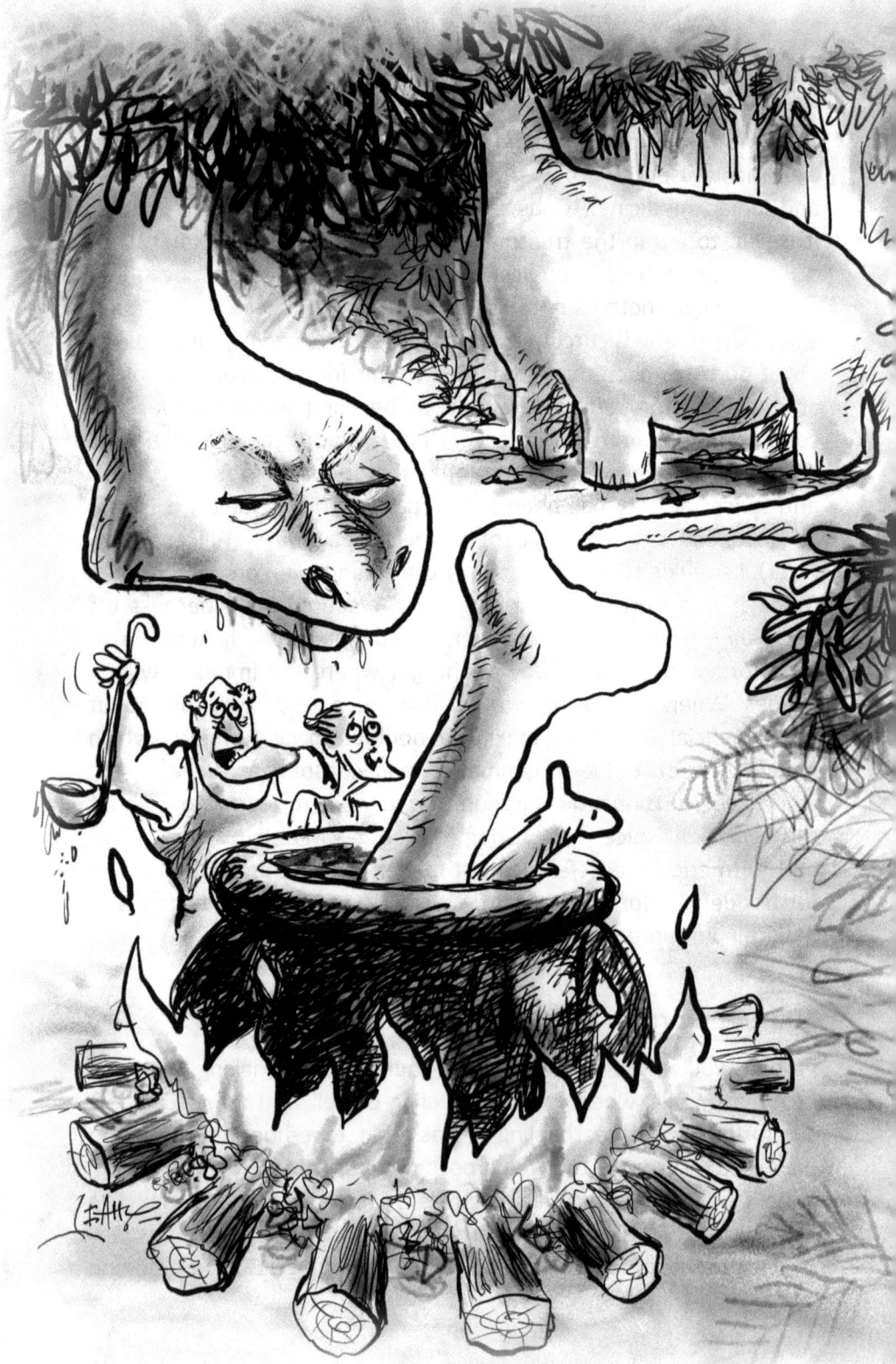

of consuming bone broth for good health goes back to the fourth century BC when Hippocrates wrote of its merits, and even further back to pre-history. Evidence has emerged that during the Stone Age, broth was cooked in turtle shells or skins over a fire (Fallon Morrell, 2014). It appears to be the elixir for a long and healthy life, it tastes delicious and it's soul-satisfying! Bone broth is said to be one of the most nutrient-dense, healing foods for the digestion. However, there are some mere mortals among us who cannot tolerate bone broth well, which I'll outline shortly.

Nutritionist and author, Sally Fallon Morrell, says that bone broth has "been known through history and across cultures [to settle] your stomach and also your nerves" (2014). Although there are few reliable recent studies on the medicinal effects of bone broth (Butler, 2015), Fallon Morrell argues that with the long tradition behind it, the science is there too. The Weston A Price Foundation, headed by Fallon Morell, has undertaken analysis that proposes benefits of consuming bone broth in addressing inflammatory diseases, digestive disorders and dopamine levels (Moskin, 2015). Twelfth-century Jewish physician, Rabbi Moses ben Maimon (Maimonides), wrote in his treatise on the merits of chicken broth that it had therapeutic value in a range of ailments including the treatment of respiratory tract disorders (Moskin, 2015).

The broth is made primarily from animal parts (ideally, grass-fed and organic) that we'd usually toss away: bones, marrow, skin, feet, tendons, and ligaments – all of which are edible and nutrient-dense. When purchasing the ingredients for your broth, try to get a 1:1:1 ratio of bones, joints and feet for a good mix of the necessary marrow and collagen (gelatine), as joints and feet contain the most collagen.

The benefits of consuming bone broth will delight you. When you combine cartilage material, water, some tasty aromatic vegetables such as celery and carrots, herbs, and a little bit of acid such as apple cider vinegar, and then boil slowly, the process extracts compounds called glycosaminoglycans. You don't have to remember or even pronounce this term. Just know that these compounds act as growth hormones and growth serum that, for starters, are said to be marvellous for your skin. They work to repair connective tissue: farewell cellulite! The old adage that beauty begins from the inside out is true regarding bone broth. These compounds work to make your skin glow and your hair grow, they lubricate your joints and they're brilliant for your arteries and kidneys. In particular, bone broth is said to be excellent for treating leaky gut syndrome as well as boosting the immune system and assisting in overcoming food intolerances and allergies (Axe, 2018; Kroeker, 2017). If it lives up to its claims, bone broth deserves the moniker 'liquid gold' that nutritionist and anti-aging expert Dr Kellyann Petrucci (2016) has attributed to it, benefiting as it does almost every aspect of your body from your brain to your gut, your muscles to your ligaments, inside and out!

I'd like to offer two cautionary notes here from personal experience regarding preparing and drinking bone broth that my initial research had not uncovered. Firstly, if using beef or pork bones and cooking for an extended period, be mindful that there may be a rather strong odour emitted from the pot. And for one who lives in a subtropical climate, I had the added visitation of flies drawn to and intoxicated by the aroma (despite the house being sealed and screened). To avoid these problems, you can use lamb or chicken bones whose odour is much milder, and you can reduce the cooking time to resolve the problem (Paleohacks, 2014). My second note, again, comes from personal experience. Occasionally, some people have an initial intolerance to the collagen and glutamic acid produced from bone broth, experiencing a reaction described as 'histamine intolerance'. Histamine is a component that is ideally designed to break down your stomach acid which in turn breaks down the food in your stomach. If you are histamine intolerant or experience any adverse reactions to the broth, then in the first instance it's best to cease taking the broth and check in with your health professional. It's also important that you give your gut time to recover before reintroducing the broth. The best way to overcome the 'problem' is by reducing the cooking time by about two-thirds. This way the levels of glutamic acid and histamine will be markedly reduced, while still allowing you to derive the benefits of this amazing food. Starting with a chicken (rather than beef) bone broth and drinking smaller portions initially are also a gentler way to ease you in (Corrado, 2015; Petrucci, 2017).

Now, assuming you're good to go, conventional bone broth is cooked long and slowly, allowing the ingredients to release their stored nutrients. Below is a recommended recipe for a slow cooker style beef bone broth (Nunes, 2018). There are also great recipes online for pressure cooker versions where you can reduce cooking time down to three hours with the same result:

Ingredients:
2 kg (4.5 lb) beef bones (marrow, knuckle and meat bones – organic, grass-fed preferably). Chicken, fish or lamb are alternatives
6 sprigs thyme
2 tbsp apple cider vinegar
2 carrots, quartered (add sweetness to the deeply savoury nature of the broth)
1 brown onion, halved
2 stalks celery, chopped
1 bay leaf
Water

Method:
1. Preheat oven (200° Celsius; 180° Celsius fan forced; 390° or 350° Fahrenheit fan forced). Roast bones for 30-60 minutes.
2. Transfer bones, fat and any other crisped brown bits to a 6-litre (1½ gallon) slow cooker with remaining ingredients and enough water to cover bones. Close lid and bring to the boil for about 20 minutes*, then on low for 24–48 hours. You should end up with a jelly-like consistency. If not, in most cases it's probably because you just need to let it simmer for longer to release the gelatine.

3. Strain into a large bowl. Cool *as quickly as possible* by placing the bowl in a sink or large tub filled with iced water. Chill. (Some even suggest putting a cup of ice cubes in the broth, which won't drastically dilute the intense flavour.) Discard the hard layer of fat.

* It's important to bring the broth to the boil for at least 20 minutes to release the collagen from the bones, so perhaps boil the water then pour it into the slow cooker rather than allowing it to come to the boil.

For more tips on making bone broth, visit Steph Gaudreau's website Bone Broth 101: How to Make the Best Bone Broth Recipe (Gaudreau, nd). It's recommended that you drink a cup of bone broth every day for several weeks. The bone broth can be kept in the refrigerator for up to five days. If you make a large enough batch, you can freeze what you don't drink. I hope you enjoy this 'liquid gold' as a means to a longer, healthier life.

20. Go nuts

I've mentioned nuts in passing elsewhere in these pages, but they deserve a little more attention because of their valuable contribution to our health and longevity, despite the small serving required to do the job. Recent studies have suggested that eating just a handful of nuts each day has the potential to lower the risk of heart disease, respiratory disease, obesity, cancer, and premature death. Around 20 g (¾ oz) per day of a range of nuts, including pecans, hazel nuts, walnuts, as well as peanuts (which are in fact legumes) have been associated, for instance, with an almost 50% reduction in respiratory disease (asthma, bronchitis, allergies and the like), and a 40% reduction in diabetes (NDTV, 2016). "We found that people who ate nuts every day lived longer, healthier lives than people who didn't eat nuts," said Dr Frank Hu, Professor of Nutrition and Epidemiology at the Harvard School of Public Health (Corliss, 2013).

Dr Fred Kummerow, a German-born biochemist whose typical diet included a handful of walnuts, pecans or almonds daily (Peat,

2015), passed away in 2017 aged 102. Kummerow is one of many thousands attesting to the benefits of nuts. Twenty-nine published studies were analysed from across the globe involving 819,000 participants, with consistent results revealing an association between nut consumption and improved health outcomes. The results were published in the *BMC Medicine Journal* (Corliss, 2013).

What's the little nut's secret? you might be asking. They're packed with antioxidants – you know, that lovely substance that inhibits oxidative stress and has the potential to reduce the risk of cancer. Nuts and peanuts are also crammed full of fibre, magnesium and polyunsaturated (good) fats – all brilliant at reducing the risk of cardiovascular disease and helping reduce cholesterol levels. Eating nuts lowers your LDL (read 'bad' cholesterol) and raises your HDL (read 'good' cholesterol). The elevated HDL then works to boost a process called 'reverse cholesterol transport', sweeping away fatty plaque from clogged arteries, this according to Dr Penny Kris-Etherton, Professor of Medicine at the University of Pennsylvania (Corliss, 2013). Despite being quite high in fat (again, good fat) there is evidence to suggest that they may reduce the risk of obesity over time because they're high in protein and fibre, which delay absorption and decrease hunger (NDTV, 2016; Corliss, 2013). I'm conscious of budgeting for good health so while nuts might seem more expensive than other snack foods, that's because they're advertised as a price per kilo, rather than by the small pack.

My September 2018 pricing on nuts in the fresh produce section of a leading Australian supermarket reveals between $20 and $35 per kg (~$2.75 per 100 g), whereas muesli and protein bars range from $13 to $69 per kg (~$4.10 per 100 g) and potato crisps $11 to $44 (~$3.30 per 100 g). Besides, you only need a handful of nuts to feel satisfied. Now, isn't that something to go nuts about?

21. Eating fewer carbs

Finally she's talking carbs, you might be thinking! There's been lots of discussion more recently in health and media circles about whether to carb or not to carb! In my opinion, it's not an either/or dilemma, but an issue around the quantity and quality of carbs. It's first important to distinguish the good from the bad. As you may already know, not all carbs are created equal. I'm not suggesting you *cut out* the carbs, but simply *cut down* on the not-so-healthy ones. The carb dilemma is both complex and simple. You've got complex carbohydrates which are made up of whole foods containing fibre and nutrients, such as fruit, vegetables, whole grains, and legumes (e.g. beans, peas and lentils). Then there's simple carbs that are wholefoods but contain no fibre, including molasses, maple syrup, fruit juice, and honey. And finally there's the refined carbohydrates which were once wholefoods but have been stripped of their fibre and nutrients. You'll recognise these as white bread, white rice, sugars, and other processed foods (Fitzgibbon, 2014; Frey, 2018).

It's a no-brainer to suggest that the simple and refined carbo-hydrates are the ones to avoid – or at the very least, cut down on. Now that we've got that sorted, let's look at why we need to eat fewer of these carbs. In 2017, the Australian scientific research body Commonwealth Scientific and Industrial Research Organisation (CSIRO) launched their low-carb diet which advocated healthy fats and vegetables and markedly reducing carbs as a means of addressing the obesity epidemic and type 2 diabetes. I've mentioned type 2 diabetes elsewhere several times, but it's worth repeating here. Type 2 diabetes is a chronic metabolic disorder where the body can't process sugar effectively due to insufficient insulin (aka insulin resistance). The severe consequences of this disease, if left untreated, are heart disease, organ damage, amputation, and loss of sight and hearing. The authors of the diet, Professor Grant Brinkworth and dietitian Pennie Taylor, undertook a one-year study of 115 people with type 2 diabetes, dividing them into two groups: those on a controlled low-carb diet, the other group on a controlled high-carb diet, but with each group consuming the same number of kilojoules each day. While both groups, on average, lost 10% of their body weight, had improvements in blood pressure levels, reduced the bad-cholesterol (LDL) levels, and experienced more stable glucose levels, it was the low-carb group that had the most significant improvements. They realised a 40% drop in their diabetes medications, a percentage twice that of the high-carb group (Graham, 2017). Here, the low-carb diet addressed the symptoms of type 2 diabetes. As you'll notice, what the CSIRO low-carb approach does is promote healthy fats and vegetables, while encouraging a reduction in carbohydrates. Here's what their daily food pyramid suggestions consist of:

Fruit and Vegetables
1 cup salad (salad leaves, capsicum, bean sprouts, tomato, herbs)
1 cup cooked greens (broccoli, asparagus, spinach, zucchini)
½ cup cooked vegetables (beans, carrots, cauliflower)
100 g (about 8) strawberries

Healthy Fats
2 tsp olive oil
60 g almonds, cashews, pecans or walnuts (two handfuls)
½ an avocado

Dairy
200 ml skimmed milk
40 g cheddar cheese (about two slices)

Protein
Two eggs
75 g chicken (about half a breast)
75 g fish (about half a fillet)

Melanie McGrice of The Dietitians Association of Australia (in Graham, 2017) cautions that this program is not for everyone due to variations in people's metabolisms, weight-loss goals, age, and whether they are emotional eaters. While acknowledging that a shift from your regular high-carb diet might be challenging at first, I believe it is well worth pursuing, especially if you're faced with type 2 diabetes and its grim health consequences. Nevertheless, guidance from your health practitioner, and support from a counsellor or health coach if your eating is triggered by emotions, would be a valuable complement to a healthier, lower-carb eating plan.

Luigi Conaro, a medieval nobleman believed to have lived beyond 100 years, wrote a treatise when aged 83 which outlined sure and certain methods for attaining a long life. Among them was his belief that 12 oz (350 g) of solid food a day was all that was required to stay hale and hearty. Similarly, Walter Breuning, who lived to the ripe old age of 114, professed that he pushed back from the table while still hungry and ate only breakfast and lunch (Jaminet, 2010). While I'm not promoting meagre eating, I do believe that when you're eating good quality nutritious food, you'll find you become satiated more readily than with vacuous empty calories in the form of simple and refined carbohydrates.

22. Ensure you have adequate coenzymeQ10

CoQ10, as it's more commonly known, is a vitamin-like substance naturally occurring in the body that is a powerful antioxidant and food-to-energy converter. It's essential in supporting the health of the heart, retarding the aging process, improving energy production in cells, preventing blood clot formation, and neutralising free radicals that oxidise blood cells (Quigley, 2017). Sadly, the aging process together with environmental toxins, chemicals, pollutants, and a poor diet all deplete us of this important substance. Master herbalist and pharmacist, Gerard Quigley (2017), says that prescription medications such as beta-blockers and cholesterol-reducing medicines disrupt the enzyme essential for the natural production of CoQ10 in the liver. And without adequate CoQ10, our physical beauty can be compromised. Weaver (2013: 99-100) says that premature aging through lack of CoQ10 is analogous to metals that oxidise and rust. Like metals, humans oxidise and age, leading to wrinkly and leathery skin. This vitamin, therefore, is a real boon to our physical appearance. And it follows that too much oxidation can also lead to disease. To prevent this 'rusting' process, we can include fish, brown rice and organ meats such as liver, heart and kidney in our diet. I eat fish regularly, but I have to be honest, I don't eat sufficient organ meats. So I take CoQ10 in supplement form. Health coach Dr Thomas Bige encourages the inclusion of CoQ10 and suggests it be taken immediately after exercise to get the maximum benefits for heart health when the heart rate is elevated (personal communication, 5 February, 2016).

Rusting our way to 100 is not an ideal way to get there. Let's stay energised and rust-free through sufficient intake of CoQ10.

23. The importance of zinc and copper

Zinc and copper are both essential minerals for the health of our bodies. Zinc is found in cells throughout the body. It's needed for the body's defence system. It's also important for cell division, cell growth, the healing of wounds, and the breakdown of carbohydrates. Your senses of smell and taste are derived from your levels of zinc. Copper's job is to help form red blood cells, and keep the blood vessels, nerves, immune system, and bones healthy. Both minerals, according to health coach Bige, are natural cancer fighters (personal communication, 5 February, 2016).

I have focused on these two minerals because I've learned that they work in tandem. One balances out the other and the absence or excess of one or the other can cause health problems. According to Dr Lawrence Wilson, a US-based nutritionist who focuses on nutritional balance, there's a copper overload in our systems (in Yabsley, 2017: 4-5). Wilson argues that the causes are several-fold. We're taking supplements that contain too much copper which leads to a zinc–copper imbalance. Zinc competes with copper in our bodies for absorption, but with so many of us deficient in zinc due to poor soil composition (if any mineral is absent in our soils, then it's deficient in our fruits and vegetables), copper dominates and accumulates. This can lead to symptoms such as lethargy, anxiety, mood swings, sleeplessness, and weight gain among other things. Processed foods and a trend towards vegetarianism (zinc is primarily found in oysters and red meat, although beans and legumes are good plant-based sources) are also factors in zinc deficiencies. A lack of magnesium (another mineral deficient in our soils) and drinking from copper pipes all lead to an accumulation of copper.

So it seems we've got too little zinc and too much copper! Wilson highly recommends we check in with a GP or other healthcare professional interested in nutritional health to determine our levels of both. Drinking filtered water and eating foods that give us a zinc/copper balance help support the removal of excess copper. A diet that includes lamb, pork, poultry, soy milk, seeds, dried beans, and wheat germ would be ideal to maintain the balance between these two important minerals (Wilson in Yabsley, 2017: 4). Bige recommends alternative days of copper and zinc. He says zinc should be taken on an empty stomach: it cleans the kidneys and then the bloodstream. Put half a teaspoon in water, mix with a non-metal spoon (metal diminishes the efficacy of the zinc) and let it sit for 15 minutes before drinking.

24. Fermented foods are fabulous

Hippocrates (460–370BC), said that "all disease begins in the gut". I've mentioned this ancient Greek physician elsewhere and I have a great deal of respect for his wisdom: it makes perfect sense that if we've got good gut health, our overall wellbeing is more likely to be maintained. There are said to be 3–4 kg of bacteria residing in the large intestine, and a fine balance of these microbes is required to ensure good health (Weaver, 2016b: 160). Good health includes a well-functioning immune system, emotional balance and the ability of the body to burn fat as fuel, to name a few. Our modern lifestyles of refined sugars and starches, stresses, antibiotics, and so on can cause the fine balance of microorganisms to be destroyed or diminished. Once that happens, we are susceptible to disease.

This is where fermented foods such as kefir, sauerkraut, yoghurt, kombucha, miso, and tempeh come in to help save the day (and your gut flora). They offer valuable probiotics that increase the levels of good bacteria in your gut. And you might be pleasantly surprised to know that fermented foods enhance your mental wellbeing.

According to Selhub *et al* (2014), there is emerging research to suggest that the consumption of fermented foods acts on the human microbiome to improve mental health. The argument here is that inflammation and oxidative stress in the gut are controlled by microbiota. The nutrients and phytochemical content of our food are enhanced and amplified by these friendly fermented foods, leading to a curbing of social anxiety and thus improved mental health. Fermenting converts glucose, fructose and sucrose (sugars) into cellular energy and lactic acid, which in turn produces digestive enzymes and healthy gut flora and cuts the sugar content in foods. The micronutrients of food are enhanced because they're full of probiotics, enzymes, vitamins, and minerals (Wilson, 2014).

A summary of the benefits of fermented foods for healthy gut: restoration of gut health, removal of toxins from the body, dramatic reduction in the sugar content of foods, rich in vitamin K2 which is said to have cancer-fighting properties, aiding the absorption of nutrients, improved mental health, and supporting the immune system. Oh, just one thing about yoghurts – so you don't compromise on the benefits of this fantastic fermented food, make sure you choose a low-sugar variety that's pot-set – yoghurt that's transferred directly to the pot to set, negating the need for thickeners or stabilisers. On her website, Sarah Wilson of *I Quit Sugar* fame has excellent recipes for sauerkraut and fermented kombucha for those who prefer to make rather than buy this wonder food (Wilson, 2014 & nd).

To minimise your risk of disease and elevate your mental wellbeing, why not trot down to your local supermarket and purchase some sauerkraut. Better still, if you've got friends or family who know how to prepare it, ask them to cook you up a batch and teach you how to make it.

25. Cook with ghee as another simple way to stay healthy

You may or may not know about the smoke point: when cooking with oils, the temperature at which an oil will smoke and burn. Low smoke point oils should be avoided for high-heat cooking, while high smoke point oils should be embraced for cooking. What this means is that the many essential nutrients and phytochemicals found in unrefined oils are destroyed when overheated. But the biggie in terms of being detrimental to your health is that oils heated past their smoke point generate toxic fumes and free radicals that in turn generate inflammation: a harmful situation for your body.

Look for an oil with a healthy balance of omega-3 to omega-6 fatty acids. Avoid low smoke point oils for cooking, including unrefined sunflower (107°C/224°F), corn (160°C/320°F), unrefined peanut (160°C/320°F), soybean (160°C/320°F), coconut (177°C/350.6°), and canola (204°C/400°F) when cooking on high heat. Even some extra-virgin olive oils with a smoke point of just 160°C (350°F) should be kept for salad dressings.

At the other end of the spectrum are the high smoke point oils such as rice bran (254°C/489°F) and avocado (271°C/520°F), along with ghee (clarified butter) (252°C/450°F). Health coach Dr Thomas Bige encourages cooking with ghee because it's rich in fat-soluble vitamins A, D and E. Ghee is also a great source of conjugated linoleic acid if it is derived from grass-fed cows. This fatty acid is known to protect against carcinogens, artery plaque and diabetes. It's also suitable for those with lactose and casein sensitivities. Another fabulous benefit to cooking with ghee is that it's rich in butyrate, a short-chain fatty acid produced in the gut that provides nutrients for your colon and reduces the risks of inflammation. On top of all that, ghee tastes even better than butter, so give ghee a go. It can be found in your supermarket or from most Indian grocery stores. If you're keen to make your own, you can find a recipe on The Pioneer Woman's website (2017).

26. Eat eggs daily

The humble egg has seen a resurgence in more recent times and thankfully so. Once upon a time, eggs were mistakenly associated with contributing to increased cholesterol levels, and thus a risk of

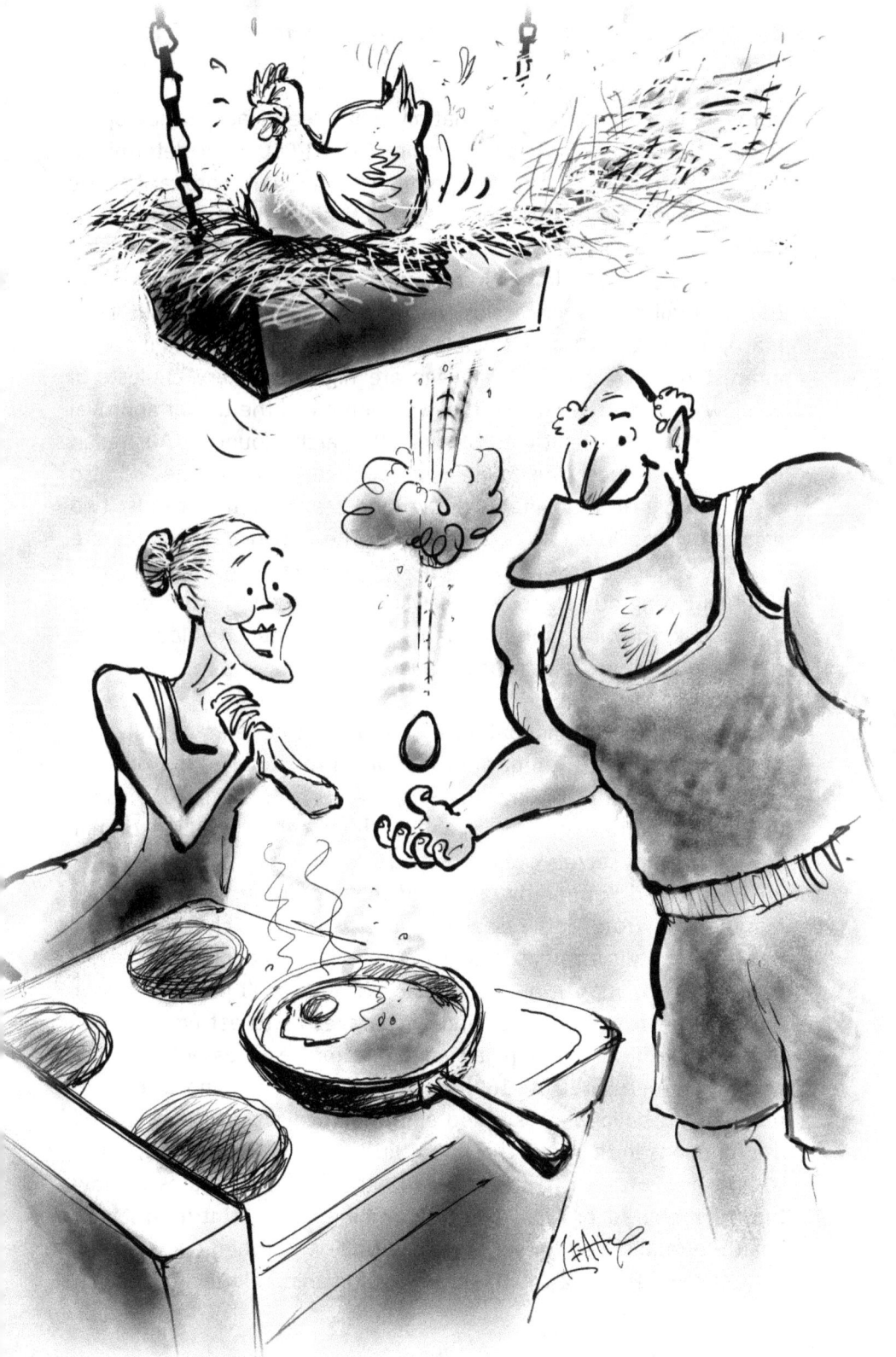

coronary heart disease. Well, that myth has been cracked wide open. A 2016 Finnish study involving more than 1,000 men determined that cholesterol or egg intake is not associated with coronary artery disease, even for those who are genetically predisposed to high blood cholesterol (Drayer, 2017). In fact, eggs are a nutrient-rich food containing 11 vitamins and minerals. They're high in protein, providing all nine amino acids that our own bodies need but can't make, building muscle and aiding satiety. That's good news if you're interested in weight control. Eggs are high in dietary cholesterol but low in saturated fats, so they've been given the tick of approval in the National Health & Medical Research Council's Australian Dietary Guidelines (Australian Eggs Limited, 2018a). They're also a rich source of antioxidants (lutein and zeaxanthin), with just two eggs providing 530 micrograms (mcg). These two antioxidants are absorbed more efficiently into the body via egg consumption than through eating other good sources such as spinach or corn because in egg yolk, they are more efficiently absorbed into the bloodstream than through vegetables (Abdel-Aal *et al,* 2013).

But the biggest commendation for the health benefits of daily egg intake has to go to Emma Morano who lived to the ripe old age of 117 years and 137 days, passing away on 15 April 2017. Born in Piedmont, Italy, her life spanned three centuries. One of her key nutritional secrets was a diet of raw eggs each day (Donato, 2016). Dr Fred Kummerow also said that he ate an egg every day. Kummerow wrote and researched extensively on cholesterol *not* being the culprit for heart disease. While acknowledging that plant-based proteins supply the nine amino acids we can't produce on our own, Kummerow recognises and encourages us to eat eggs as part of our daily diet to ensure an adequate intake of essential amino acids (Kummerow, 2014: 169). Kummerow said, "amino acids [are required] to build what is called endothelin cells, and they carry all the functions in the body that cause life" (Here & Now, 2014). There is, however, a caveat with regard to eggs, and that relates to how they're prepared or what they're combined with. Nutritionist and health journalist Lisa Drayer says that while a poached egg contains only 71 calories and 2 g (0.07 oz) of fat, and an omelette and spinach using the yolk is also a lean choice, there are high calories at stake with the likes of eggs benedict with its hollandaise sauce and side of bacon: hello 800 calories and 26 g (0.9 oz) of fat. Drayer (2017) advocates balancing egg intake with fibre-rich foods such as fruits, vegetables and whole grains. So egg up because they're egg-ceptional. I'm not yolking!

27. Milk matters

Some of my readers might recall a tradition at school during the 50s, 60s and 70s where we'd all file out onto the footpath at 'little lunch' (morning break around 10 am) after the dairy produce trucks had dumped crates of silver-capped bottles of milk in the early hours of the morning for our mandated consumption. With Queensland summers reaching 37.7°C (100°F) for several months of the year and large-scale refrigeration for schools still a distant thought bubble, the milk would invariably be lukewarm at best or cringingly curdled at worst. There was no escaping the line, with the 'milk monitors' ensuring we downed the whole bottle before returning the empty to the crate. Known as the School Milk Program, the theory was that every Australian child was considered healthier with a daily dairy dose and a calcium boost. While the program's intentions were commendable, some of you may have been scarred for life because of the experience, either because of the 'yuck factor' or more disturbingly, a lactose allergy.

Despite the grim picture I've painted, it needs to be said that milk has since had an important revival, so I'd like to help you reimagine its merits to enjoy the taste and know that it punches well above its weight in the health stakes. If you haven't touched the stuff since that milk-menacing time, please do hang in there with me, but if you're milk intolerant or have made a conscious decision not to consume dairy for whatever reason, I perfectly understand your diffidence. Nevertheless, I do offer some very important alternatives to milk that will hopefully provide the essential (and in some cases, vital) nutrients found in this food source. In the meantime, for the milk lovers and potential converts among you,

you'll be pleased to know that milk is not only excellent for your physical health but also the intellect (more on this later). Known in the pastoral economy of New Zealand as 'liquid gold', this protein is an excellent source of calcium to counter osteoporosis. For instance, the vitamin D found in milk is brilliant for bones, muscles and cell regeneration and as a protection against cancer. Potassium is also found in milk, a nutrient said to reduce blood pressure and the risks associated with cardiovascular disease. Milk is also rich in vitamin B12 and phosphorous (Department of Health & Human Services, 2013a). More significantly, cow's milk is a source of iodine. It's an essential trace element imperative for the production of thyroxine, a hormone that controls our metabolic rate (Nutrition Australia, 2010). Insufficient levels of iodine can lead to a slowing of our metabolism, weight gain and unpredictable mood swings (Mosley, 2018). Wait: so drinking milk can actually help us lose weight and lift our spirits? No wonder the Kiwis call it liquid gold! Alongside these physical and emotional benefits is the connection to an enhanced intellect. An iodine deficiency was once linked to cretinism, a condition characterised by severely stunted physical and mental growth (Mosley, 2018). While that is not so prevalent today, Michael Mosley (2018) reports on a United Kingdom study which found that even a mild iodine deficiency in pregnant women could significantly impact the developing brain of their unborn baby. This study looked at the IQ and reading ability of these children when aged nine and noted their lower scores when compared with those children born to mothers with adequate iodine levels. The World Health Organization (WHO) has discovered that communities with low iodine levels have an IQ score that is 13 points lower than iodine-sufficient populations. Australia has a mild, but still concerning, iodine deficiency overall (The Australian Thyroid Foundation Ltd, 2018), this compared with 70% of Britain's teenage female population with levels below the WHO recommendations (Mosley, 2018). It's important to note too that iodine is vital to breast health. Dr Libby Weaver (2013: 182) tells us that the breasts (and ovaries) concentrate iodine but a deficiency of this element can produce a form of oestrogen linked to breast cancer. Another important reason to get your iodine sources wherever you can. To avoid cow's milk, many people have switched to non-dairy forms derived from soya, coconut, almonds, and oats. However, these alternatives lack the necessary levels of iodine, with one study at the University of Surrey finding these sources contained just 2% of the iodine found in cow's milk. If, however, you really can't stomach milk, you're lactose intolerant, vegan, or have made a conscious decision not to drink milk for any number of valid reasons, then there are other sources that are relatively rich in iodine. Many of our breads are now fortified with iodine, and white fish and seaweed have been recommended as great alternatives. However, when Michael Mosley, in association with Glasgow University, tested 12 volunteers over 12 days, comparing their iodine levels across white fish, seaweed and milk, it was found that volunteers consuming the seaweed absorbed only about half the levels derived from fish and milk. As a fibrous food, it seems our bodies struggle to break seaweed down to absorb sufficient iodine, and the levels in the range of seaweeds vary greatly. I mention this because some may rely on seaweed as a main source of this trace element and will need to take this variability and unpredictability into consideration. For those who choose to drink cow's milk, it's recommended that we have 150 mcg per day for adults and 200 mcg for pregnant and lactating women. To put that into perspective, one glass of milk can provide up to 100 mcg of iodine (Hobson, 2017).

I've just about milked this topic for all it's worth, but my hope is that you'll consider milk as a healthy food source because for many of us, there's nothing the matter with milk.

28. Salt and you

Writer, poet and visual artist Khalil Gibran (1883–1931) once wrote that "there must be something sacred in salt. It is in our tears and in the ocean". Salt is a substance that has long been associated with life itself, and our physiology depends on the important balance of salts and liquids. When out of balance, disease may follow. The ancient Egyptians and Greeks knew of its significance as a medical treatment. Hippocrates, 2,500 years ago, utilised unrefined sea salt for the healing of skin lesions, advocated drinking salty or mineralised water for digestive disorders and recommended inhaling salt for respiratory complaints (Wormer, 1999). The ancients didn't have the overconsumption problems of processed table salt that we have today, or our propensity for packaged and processed foods. Seventy-five per cent of the average Australian's salt intake is derived this processed way each day. In Australia, it's recommended that daily, we eat less than 5 g of salt (less than 1 tsp, 2,000 mg of sodium) (National Heart Foundation of Australia, nd). If you're primarily eating loads of unprocessed and real/raw foods, then you'll want to ensure you have an adequate intake of a quality salt. Aside from being a natural flavouring, salt has important benefits in promoting health. Ideal salts include Celtic sea salt (grey coloured) and Himalayan rock salt (pink), both of which are rich in trace minerals. Himalayan rock salt is sourced from the Punjab region close to the Himalayan Mountains, the salt fields there dating back some four billion years. Celtic sea salt, comparable to its Himalayan cousin, is sourced from Brittany in France and contains around 60 mineral elements. These essential salts support hydration and fluid balance, the theory being that when the body is low in sodium, water loss occurs leading to dehydration and thirst. Adequate good quality salt intake allows for an equilibrium of electrolytes (sodium and potassium) ensuring balance across the body's cells, blood plasma and extracellular fluid. The major electrolytes of sodium, magnesium, calcium, and potassium are important for regulating the heartbeat and allowing for muscle contractions: an imbalance in these can have life-threatening consequences. But wait, there's even more benefits to good salt intake. Sodium is an important transmitter of electrical signals in the body, enabling appropriate brain, muscle and nervous system functioning. Digestive health is also improved, with sufficient salt in the diet producing the ever-important hydrochloric acid (HCL) for food digestion. Finally, by having sufficient stomach acid, you're better able to absorb the calcium, zinc, iron, folate, and B12 minerals (Axe, 2018a). As Himalayan rock salt and Celtic salt contain minimal iodine, if you're iodine deficient, then you may need to source your iodine elsewhere such as from iodised salt, seafood such as shellfish or tinned salmon, pre-packaged breads, or dairy foods (Nutrition Australia, 2010).

You're probably wondering how to calculate if you're getting sufficient or too much salt in your diet. If you're consuming pre-packaged foods then a good litmus test is to look at the food label for the amount of salt: if a 100 g serving is more than 5 g of salt (0.6 g sodium), then this is considered a high salt content. Conversely, a 100 g serving with less than 0.3 g (0.1 g sodium) is considered low (Organic Facts, 2017). It pays to calculate your salt intake to make sure you're not going over the recommended intake. Salt is a fundamental aspect of the human condition and good quality salt, used in moderation, is considered one of the good guys for our health and longevity. In borrowing a biblical expression, you could say it's the 'salt of the earth'.

29. Go fish

If there's a food that could be labelled 'honest to goodness', then fish (especially fish low in mercury) has to be it. Fish has been identified as one of the healthiest foods on the planet. While no single topic in this book provides the 'silver bullet' to longevity, consuming marine food would have to be as close as you can get. Fish, especially fatty fish, is a high-quality protein packed full of omega-3 fatty acids DHA (docosahexaenoic), EPA (eicosapentaenoic acid) and DPA (docosapentaenoic acid), along with vitamins D and B2. Fish is also a rich source of calcium and phosphorous alongside minerals such as iron, zinc, iodine, magnesium, and potassium. Aside from all this nutrient data, what makes fish so fabulous? Our bodies can't produce these essential nutrients, so we must source them from the foods we eat. Fatty fish is a very important source. And if that doesn't get you into a fish frenzy, then perhaps you'll be excited by the fact that we need them to keep our brain and heart ticking along nicely. The fish families I'm talking about include salmon, trout, sardines, herring, canned mackerel, canned light tuna, and oysters (Department of Health & Human Services, Victorian Government, 2013). Fish is versatile too: you can bake it, steam it, poach it, grill it,

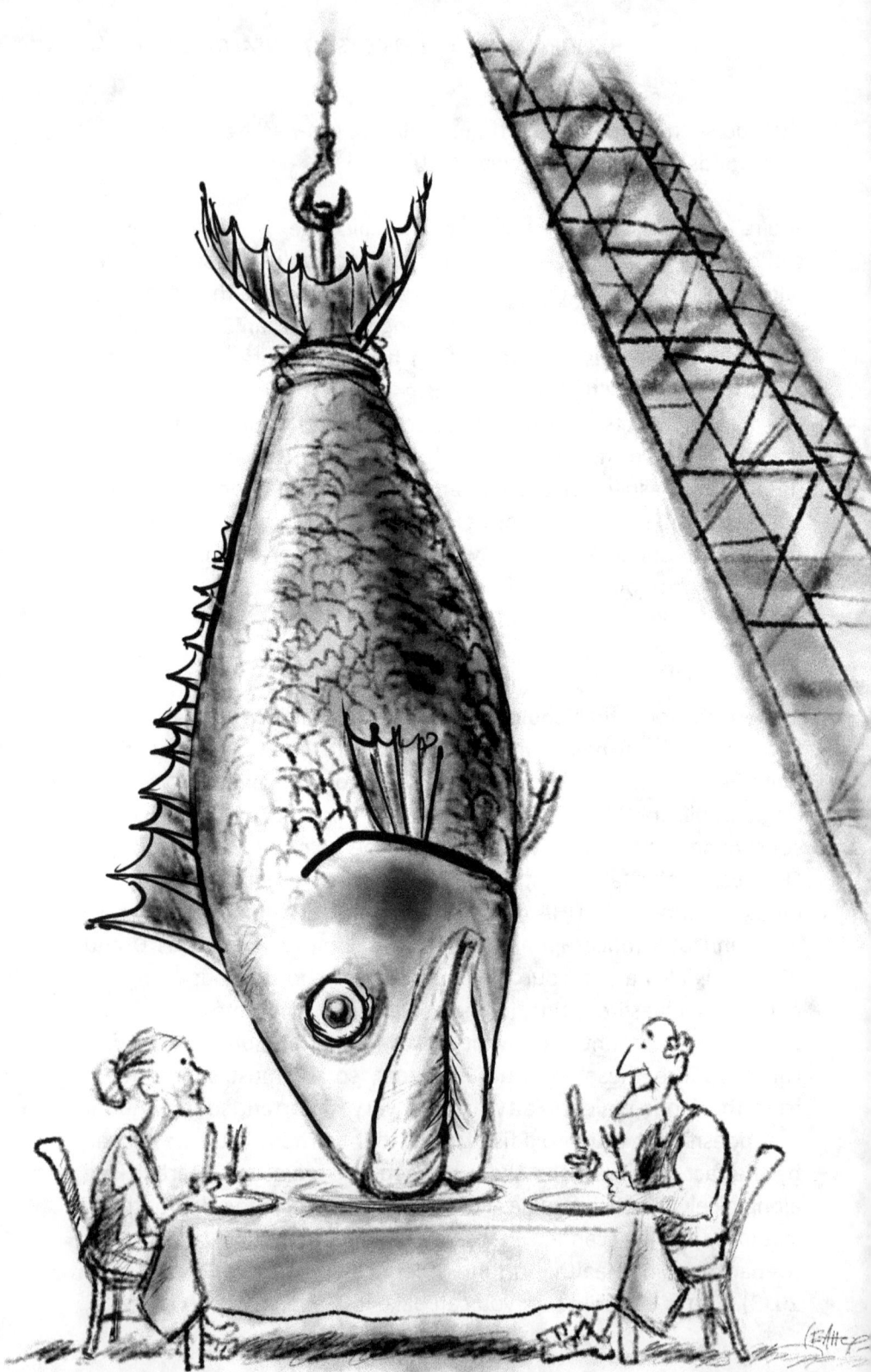

turn it into patties, barbeque it, and it goes with just about any side dish. Having two to three fish meals per week is said to lower your blood pressure, and reduce your risk of heart attack, arrhythmia and stroke. Your brain will be eternally grateful with the enhanced brain function that is a consequence of consuming omega-3. The reasoning behind this is that 60% of the brain is composed of DHA and EPA. Cultures such as the Inuit, whose diet is rich in DHA, have a lower incidence of multiple sclerosis (MS), a degenerative disease of the central nervous system (Juan, 2006). Pregnant women will be supporting the development of their unborn baby's vision and nervous system. There's also the potential for reducing the risk of depression, ADHD, Alzheimer's disease, dementia, and diabetes. Meanwhile, if arthritis is your nemesis then our friendly fish will have you hooked because of its potential for preventing inflammation (Leech, 2015).

Now, before you get too carried away considering membership at Mensa with the extra brain power you'll be harnessing, Dr Shaw Somerset of Griffith University has told us that no studies have yet proven that eating more fish will give you the smarts. Nevertheless, consuming fatty fish regularly certainly provides the foundation for good health, and dare I say, a fountain of youth as the following might attest. In a 16-year study of 2,700 healthy adults aged over 65, those with higher levels of all three fatty acids had a 35% lower risk of death compared to those with lower levels in their blood, and the higher fatty-acid group lived, on average, more than two years longer (Sifferlin, 2013). The Japanese people in Okinawa, whom I've written about elsewhere in the book, have a diet that is also rich in fish. The Okinawans have the largest proportion of supercentenarians in the country and the oldest demographic in the world. Gerontologist and researcher of The Okinawa Program, Dr Craig Wilcox, has come to appreciate the secret to their longevity which he says is "to eat as low down the food chain as possible" (Booth, 2013), and fatty fish in its natural state is about as far from processed food as you can get. So, go fish!

30. Frypans: non-stick, cast iron or stainless steel?

I use a frypan every morning and until I began researching the benefits or otherwise of non-stick (Teflon and Calphalon) cookware, I wasn't aware of the potential safety concerns. So I did a little digging, and this is what I discovered. Canadian scientists Bruce Lourie and Rick Smith (2013) warned against using non-stick frypans. As part of their experiment in a controlled environment, the scientists released a small bird into the same room in which they heated a non-stick frypan. Within moments, the bird fell to the ground, its tiny respiratory system having suffered from polymer fume fever when overcome by the chemical polytetrafluoroethylene (PTFE). I'd like to be able to tell you that the bird survived, but I'm sorry to say that the scientists didn't elaborate on that. This story is akin to the canary in a coalmine where the canary's demise indicated the presence of deadly gases. The small bird's collapse in the controlled environment alerted the two scientists to the toxins emitted by the heated cookware. Non-stick pans are meant to be safe for humans as long as the heat doesn't exceed 200°C (~500°F) which equates to a medium heat on some cooktops. Additionally, if the coating on the non-stick pan breaks down, surface particles and/or toxic gases are released (Corriher, nd). So, for the good of my health, I don't use non-stick cookware.

Safer alternatives for frypans include cast iron and stainless steel. Nutritional coach Marc Halpern (2015) presents the case for both types. He prefers the cast iron option because of the even heat distribution and because they're relatively inexpensive. However, he does caution that they may leach iron into your food. While the amounts are probably minute, for those who are iron sensitive or don't want to risk additional iron intake, the preference might be for the stainless steel variety. Quality stainless steel with a copper core is more expensive. As with cast iron, it is not non-stick so requires different cleaning and maintenance. However, they're scratch resistant and don't create a chemical reaction with the food (Paleo Leap, 2017). So it would seem that for that extra health benefit, cooking with good quality cookware is the way to fry the fat.

31. Mind your eating

Do you ever recall your parents or grandparents telling you to 'chew your food well'? I remember it being particularly difficult to do, especially if I was hungry and more so if the food was mouth-wateringly delicious. But there is definite wisdom in the adage. I also recall many times consuming food while busy doing other things (on the phone, watching television, working) without a second thought to taking my time or appreciating the food I was consuming with gusto. The buzz term today for chewing your food well is 'mindfulness eating'. There's even an International Mindful Eating Day set aside to acknowledge its importance – 26 January. Now, for many Australians, that's also a national day of acknowledgement, Australia Day, and so it's probably quite appropriate that we should be mindfully eating our barbequed lamb chops (or food of choice) as we recognise being Australian citizens. But for emotional and physical wellbeing, *every* day needs to be a mindfulness eating day.

The physical benefits of chewing food well include a healthier digestive system due to the smaller particles of food, offsetting potential digestive problems as well as aiding in gut health; the saliva that is generated from prolonged chewing generates the enzyme lingual lipase that is a whiz at breaking down fats; nutrients are absorbed more readily into the system; and slow chewing aids in maintaining a healthy weight as it provides the time for satiety (the feeling of fullness) to kick in, which means consuming fewer calories (Mercola, 2017; Weaver, 2016a).

The notion of mindfully eating goes way beyond just chewing food 30-plus times before swallowing. The philosophy around food of the Center for Mindful Eating (nd) is that there's no right or wrong in regard to our approach to food. The important consideration is to bring a degree of *awareness* to the food experience. Mindful eating allows us to reflect on our inner wisdom to discern food's nourishing and nurturing benefits. This in turn leads to using all our senses so that the foods we choose are both nourishing and satisfying. Ultimately, this philosophy helps individuals make choices that support heightened health and wellbeing. If you're interested in learning more about your attitudinal approach to food, then I'd encourage you to explore this topic more fully.

32. Intermittent or short-term fasting for health and weight loss

I came to this topic reluctantly because I was conflicted over its benefits. I'd read so many arguments *against* fasting along with as many views in favour. Besides, I *love* food and I tended to shy away from the thought of denying myself this wonderful pleasure in life. Nevertheless, I worked through my prejudices and researched as objectively as I could. Early in my research, I concluded that *prolonged* fasting is a definite no-no – at least in my book. However, my findings brought me to an appreciation of the enormous benefits that can be derived from *intermittent* or *short-term* fasting. Essentially, intermittent fasting allows you to eat a normal healthy diet over specific time periods. My main source of inspiration – the giant on whose shoulders I had to stand in order to see and appreciate the merits of this form of fasting – is Dr Mark Mattson. Mattson (2018) is a neuroscientist with The University of Iowa, and the Chief of the Laboratory of Neurosciences at the National Institute on Aging in Baltimore. He is considered a leader in cellular and molecular mechanisms that underlie neurodegenerative disorders such as Alzheimer's disease, Parkinson's disease and stroke. He has decades of research to his name and has been an advocate of intermittent fasting for the past 35 years. Each time you eat, glucose is stored in the liver as glycogen and this takes up to 12 hours to deplete. Once the glycogen stores are exhausted, your body begins to burn fat which is then converted into ketone bodies (acidic chemicals used by neurons as energy). These ketones stimulate positive changes in the structure of synapses in the brain that are important for learning, memory and overall brain health. However, when you eat three meals a day plus snacks in between, your body doesn't get the chance to deplete the glycogen stored in your liver and the ketones aren't generated (Sugarman, 2016).

Clinical trials have shown that intermittent fasting leads to weight loss, improved blood sugar levels and a decrease in the risks associated with heart disease and cancer. Mattson's research suggests intermittent fasting prevents Alzheimer's and Parkinson's and improves mood and memory (Young, 2018). The benefits of intermittent fasting equate to a healthier heart, a lowering of LDL (bad) cholesterol by up to 32% and an improvement in blood pressure. There'll be a drop in your body fat (not just your overall weight) and you'll better control your blood sugars because you won't be craving that sugar fix. Studies on intermittent fasting have shown that the body's sensitivity to insulin (the hormone that regulates sugar) is increased, giving you protection against type 2 diabetes. You'll be better placed to fight fatty liver disease because fasting activates proteins that control the absorption of fatty acids into the liver. From an aesthetic perspective, you'll be warding off those wrinkles, fine lines and spots that are otherwise caused by an exposure to free radicals – you know, those pesky atoms that cause damage to your cells, proteins and DNA.

While all this information sounds good, as a persistent researcher I had to know the 'how' and 'why' of it all in order to be truly convinced. Mattson provided the answers, which clinched it for me. He explained that through his research and trials he'd discovered, "nerve cells possess an innate ability to respond adaptively to intermittent challenges in ways that help them perform optimally and counteract the adversities of aging, thereby forestalling Alzheimer's and Parkinson's diseases". The 'challenges' he refers to relate to the body being subjected to intermittent fasting. This benefits our health because it poses a challenge to our cells. In turn, those cells adapt by improving their capability for stress and aiding in disease resistance (Mattson, 2015). So, when fasting intermittently or short term, our bodies switch from a 'growing old' model to a 'repair and regenerate' model. His arguments and research findings not only made sense to me but pleased me no end with their close connection to a long and healthy life.

Mattson suggests two forms of fasting. Firstly, there's what he calls the 5:2 diet which Dr Michael Mosley made famous in his documentary *Eat, Fast and Live Longer*, featuring Mattson (Mosley, 2012). This form of fasting requires restricting your calorie intake to 500 calories over two non-consecutive days each week, while having a normal healthy diet for the rest of the week (for women: 2,000 calories; for men: 2,500 calories). The second fasting strategy is a time-restricted one in which you fit all your meals of the day into an eight- to 10-hour period. Your body then has time to use up its supply of glycogen, begin burning fat and produce the necessary ketones. Mattson argues for both forms of fasting. The time-restricted approach has similar effects to those of the intermittent approach (Sugarman, 2016).

With any new regime you commence, it's wise to start slowly but to persist with it. Mattson draws an analogy with exercise: "If you've been sedentary and then all of a sudden you try to run five miles, it's not very pleasant and you'll likely get discouraged. It's the same thing as if you've been eating three meals a day plus snacks, and then you're not eating anything at all for two days; you're not going to like it" (Sugarman, 2016). The benefits of 5:2 fasting are that you can eat your normal healthy food on five of the seven days each week. You need only count calories on your fasting days. It's a well-tested, proven and safe method through human trials. It'll decrease your cholesterol, triglycerides and blood pressure. Moreover, you'll burn fat at a greater rate than any other 'diet'. Challenges associated with the 5:2 fast are that the limited calorie intake on the two days could leave you a little energy-depleted. Initial headaches and sleeplessness could arise in the first week or so, and your fasting days might interfere with your social life and/or family meal preparation. The time-restricted daily fast of 14 to 16 hours offers the opportunity to eat your normal healthy food regime within the remaining eight- to 10-hour span. There are no caloric restrictions (trials on mice showed that the time-restricted subjects lost weight even if they ate the same number of calories as the mice eating throughout the day). This fast is said to reduce inflammation and improve brain function and blood pressure. If you are able to schedule your meal window between 7 am and 5 pm, when your metabolism and blood sugar levels are at their highest, you are allowing for more effective burning of calories. On the downside, the restricted period can interfere with your social life. Eating earlier in the day is said to be most effective; however, this might be difficult to sustain with your family dynamics. Moreover, there have been no human studies conducted on this fast as yet (Graves, 2015). Fasting isn't for everyone. If you're already at below normal weight or you have a health condition that might preclude fasting, it's best to seek the guidance of your health practitioner before proceeding. That said, please see my *Reference List* for web links to the various authors mentioned in this section and beyond (Mattson (2015, 2018)); Sugarman (2016); Mosley (2012); and Graves (2015)), then make your decision to fast or not.

33. Do your sums for a healthy weight

You've probably noticed that I don't focus on losing weight *per se* in this book. Maintaining a healthy weight is often a little easier said than done. However, if you're following the nutritional and lifestyle choices discussed in these pages, then you'll more than likely be on track with your ideal weight anyway. Nevertheless, calculating where you stand in the healthy body weight stakes is a topic worth discussing because the levels of obesity evident here in Australia and many other countries around the world are frighteningly high. Historically, the primary tool for determining weight and fat status has been the BMI. In the 1970s, American physiologist Ancel Keys was credited with the name for a formula developed in the 1840s whereby you divide your weight (in kg or lb) by your height (in m or ft), then divide the answer by your height again to get your BMI. Apart from an obvious level of complexity to this system, the problem with the method is that it was introduced before the invention of the calculator, so it lacks any sense of accuracy, but more importantly it doesn't take into account abdominal fat. The amount of visceral adipose tissue located around your tummy is a gauge for your weight status as well as an indicator of several major health conditions such as cardiovascular disease, type 2 diabetes and breast cancer (MacLellan & Zhou, 2017).

Other health challenges with obesity include gallstones, asthma, cataracts, infertility, snoring, and sleep apnoea (Harvard T H Chan School of Public Health, 2018). Today there's a much more accurate (and simple) formula for determining whether you have a problem with body fat. This method is called the waist-height ratio (WHtR). Simply divide your waist measurement by your height to get your result which, ideally, should equate to less than 50% for healthy people (MacLellan & Zhou, 2017). So, for a woman in her 60s with a height of 162.5 cm (5'4") and a waist circumference of 71 cm (28"), the ratio would be 44% which is within the 'healthy' range. If you don't have a tape measure handy, you need only use a piece of string to measure your height, then fold the string in half and check to see if it fits around your waist. Michelle Swainson, Professor of Physiology at Lancaster University in the United Kingdom, calculates that the cut-off for predicting whole body obesity in women is .54 and in men .53 (MacLellan & Zhou, 2017). If your pants are becoming tight around the waist, that's another good indicator, unless you're convinced your clothes have all shrunk in the wash! Don't despair if the WHtR or string test indicates you're overweight. Rather, use it as a wake-up call towards eating good quality foods and getting moving, both of which, in my opinion, are the two key ingredients to a healthy weight-height ratio. Don't eat too little, because all that will do is send a message to your body that you're starving yourself and your metabolism, in its infinite wisdom, will slow down to conserve your stores of fat. Avoiding being overweight by eating well was another guideline of Dr Shigeaki Hinohara, whose 105 years of life must surely be an example for us to live up to (Gillett, 2017). Sensible eating and sensible exercise are key to a healthy body weight, and to a longer life.

34. Reduce your alcohol intake

It has to be said that alcohol and good health are not synonymous. I'm no teetotaller so I'm not preaching from a pulpit on this topic.

I enjoy white wine – Pinot Gris is my current favourite. However, it's primarily the *overindulgence* of alcohol I'd like to chat about. Dr Libby Weaver (2016b; Weaver, nd) adopts a sensible approach to her discussions around alcohol. While she ideally encourages us to quit alcohol altogether, she's mindful that it's a cultural and social activity of celebration, or something we might use to wind down, but it's also a substance to treat with respect and moderation. Nevertheless, many of us overconsume alcohol with the consequent physical, emotional and social damages. Alcohol consumption can lead to body fat and cellulite, a loss of vitality and energy, mood swings, and heightened bouts of premenstrual tension (PMT), not to mention a reduction in clarity of thought. And here's another deterrent that might make you think twice about alcohol: did you know that alcohol can multiply the gas-producing bacteria in your gut by a factor of a thousand? (Enders, 2016).

Your body cannot excrete alcohol directly. Instead, the liver converts it to acetaldehyde, a poisonous substance that registers its presence through the 'hangover' we experience the next day. Such is the poisonous nature of alcohol that if our liver can't do its job effectively, the alcohol would accumulate in our blood, put us in a coma and ultimately, we could die.

On a less sinister note, let's look at some guidelines for consumption and the road to a healthier you. The Australian Heart Foundation and National Health and Medical Research Council recommend no more than two standard drinks per day for both women and men (Department of Health, 2013). Weaver (nd) suggests that we also have two alcohol-free days a week. A standard drink equates to just 100 ml of liquid (or about four swallows if you need a reality check on volume). It might be worth measuring 100 ml into a glass to see whether you're drinking above the recommended two glasses.

For those with a history of cancer in the family, expert studies have revealed that they should seriously consider ceasing alcohol altogether because of the link between even light drinking and disease, especially breast cancer. While not trying to frighten you with this data, it's an opportunity to reflect on your drinking habits and consider alcohol's side effects and negative impacts on your health – physically, emotionally, socially, and psychologically. If you need support with alcohol or drug addiction, I recommend you contact the Alcohol and Drug Information Service; telephone 1800 177 833 (Australian readers).

Another great source of support is an organisation called Hello Sunday Morning (HSM). Founded in 2010, it is the largest online movement for alcohol behaviour change in the world. HSM's philosophy centres around supporting individuals to modify their relationship with alcohol. Founder, Chris Raine, recognised Saturday night as the big drinking night, with the inevitable hangover Sunday morning. Raine's philosophy is that "drinking is an individual choice, not a cultural expectation" (HSM, 2018). See my *Reference List* for the web link.

35. Cut out the caffeine

Now, for all you latte lovers, long black devotees, double-shot-cappuccino aficionados, and any-other-kinda-coffee-you-can-think-of-sorts, please do read on despite your horror at the thought of giving up your much-loved beverage. You might be surprised (or not) to learn that nearly 10 million tons of coffee is consumed each year across the globe and that Finland is the most ardent coffee-drinking country. Each Finn consumes around 9.6 kg (21.1 lb), while Aussies sip on a mere 3 kg (6.6 lb) each year (Padovese, 2017). These figures include the 'hidden' caffeine in energy and soft drinks.

While the Australian statistics might suggest we don't have a problem with caffeine when compared with Finland, caffeine has the same effect on the body as a marauding woolly mammoth would have had on early humans when confronted by their foe. Caffeine ignites the stress hormones and fires you up, activating the flight-or-fight response. Adrenalin is released, elevating your blood sugars, your blood pressure and your pulse rate (Weaver, 2013: 129). You're ready to face your fears or run for your life.

Imagine being in this state regularly – daily even – and constantly over years when consuming coffee. As Weaver points out, this biochemical state creates a situation in your body where all your resources and nutrients are directed to saving your life, shutting down any other non-vital processes. Over an extended period of caffeine consumption, there are negative consequences for these non-vital processes when denied important nutrients. What's more, the stress response elicits cortisol and increases insulin, which in turn increases inflammation in the body. As I've mentioned elsewhere, inflammation leads to disease (Hyman, nd). The fight/flight response, initiated by caffeine, draws on glucose (sugar), so with glucose depletion, the body requires more and craves more as a consequence. Your coffee drinking is indirectly teaching your body to crave sugar. With the additional glucose in your system, insulin is released, a fat storage hormone. Any excess will be converted to body fat. Some of the other symptoms of caffeine consumption include adrenal fatigue, increased heart rate, tremors, anxiety, elevated blood pressure, restless sleep, dulled complexion, and moodiness (Weaver, 2013: 133). We can't be certain of a correlation between caffeine consumption and increased heart disease in the Finnish community. However, the most common cause of death, associated with one-fifth of all deaths in Finland, is ischaemic heart disease. (Statistics Finland, 2015). If these figures are anything to go by, then the detriment to your health must surely outweigh the five minutes of exhilaration to your taste and olfactory senses!

In the interests of fairness and balance, I have read counter-arguments (Park, 2017) that claim caffeine is in fact good for your health and longevity. I'll outline this here but, to be honest, with a healthy scepticism. In one study published in the *Annals of Internal Medicine* (Park *et al,* 2017), 700,000 Americans and Europeans responded to a questionnaire on coffee consumption. Their findings of a three-year study (1993–1996) and a 16-year follow-up until 2012 suggest that coffee drinkers tended to live longer than their non-caffeine-drinking counterparts. However, as the researchers conceded themselves, the data for non-whites is sparse. The participants self-reported their coffee consumption, and the strength of the brew was not determined; the health benefits were reflected in decaffeinated as well as caffeinated versions, suggesting not caffeine as the longevity hero but perhaps some other component such as an antioxidant; and the researchers still cautioned consumers to limit their intake due to possible adverse side effects such as agitation, irregular heartbeat and digestive problems (Park *et al*, 2017).

If you're still reading, dear caffeine drinkers, and have decided that it's worth giving up your beloved brew, then there are strategies and alternatives you can try. Weaver (2013: 133) suggests that if you're experiencing any or all of the symptoms outlined earlier, that you try giving up caffeine totally for a four-week trial period. While you're 'decaffeinating', it's wise to increase your water consumption, take a good quality vitamin C supplement, indulge in some daily light exercise, and substitute the coffee for real food such as nuts or seeds like almonds, walnuts, pecans, and pumpkin seeds. Recent research by Professor Patrick O'Connor of the University of Georgia in the US has revealed that taking a 10-minute walk up and down a flight of stairs is the equivalent to the energy derived from a 50 mg standard coffee (Morales, 2017). All these strategies can assist with any withdrawal symptoms (Hyman, nd). Then there are the coffee alternatives such as Teeccino caffeine-free herbal coffee or the range of herbal teas such as green, liquorice, reishi mushroom, or rooibos.

36. Sip your way to a kidney cleanse

Our kidneys are an important filtering system for our bodies. Just as air filters get rid of dust and other allergens, our kidneys work to remove waste and other toxins from our blood. Yay to our kidneys! However, they can get overworked and they need support to keep them operating smoothly. Dr Edward Group of the Global Healing Center in Houston argues that environmental factors, urinary tract infections (UTIs), nonsteroidal anti-inflammatory drugs, and of course any processed foods we consume all put a strain on our dear, hard-working kidneys (2014). If our kidneys are not working optimally, then any waste that makes its way to our bloodstream can cause serious health concerns, so looking after them is a no-brainer.

The obvious first strategy is to drink plenty of filtered water – around 1.5 litres (see the earlier section on *Drinking water*), to quench your thirst and keep your urine colourless or light yellow. More importantly, water gives your kidneys a good flush (Group, 2014). Health coach Dr Thomas Bige especially recommends cranberry juice to reduce the risk of UTIs. Cranberries coat the bladder and ward off bacteria adhering to the bladder and urethra. Cranberries contain high levels of an antioxidant known as proanthocyanidins (PACs) which do the job nicely. And with the expected decline in UTIs with cranberry juice consumption, the *Journal of Urology* has concluded that there would be a reduction in the need for antibiotics, otherwise leading to antibiotic-resistant microorganisms (Luis, Domingues & Pereira, 2017). All this from the unassuming cranberry! Bige recommends *organic* cranberry juice. Better still, you can juice your own if they're available, with a 25/75% cranberry (50 ml) to water (200 ml) ratio. It's best to drink it anytime between 3 and 7 pm, when the kidneys are most receptive to reactivation (Bige, personal communication, 21 September 2016). Group (2014) considers cranberries useful in cleansing the kidneys of excess calcium oxalate, a major contributor to kidney stones.

Beet juice is another good source of kidney care, not just the beloved red beetroot, but also sugar beets and golden beets among others (the benefits of beetroot are extolled under the earlier heading *All you can beet: beetroot*). They contain betaine, an important phytochemical designed to ward off pathogens, and they have an antioxidant quality designed to reduce calcium phosphate build-up which would otherwise lead to kidney stones. Lemon juice (see also *Lemon juice and apple cider vinegar*) is another great kidney cleanser, with its naturally acidic state discouraging those nasty kidney stones. Finally, there's your trusted vegetable juice, giving your kidneys a welcome antioxidant and nutrient hit to facilitate toxin removal (Group, 2014).

I've avoided mentioning any more arduous kidney cleansing processes as I think it's best to check in with a health professional before proceeding down that path, especially if you are experiencing any serious kidney issues. In the meantime, enjoy these gentle and effective approaches for happy, healthy kidneys.

37. Get your daily sunshine vitamin

Vitamin D (cholecalciferol) is produced naturally in our bodies when we have sufficient exposure to the sun's rays. We can also source a percentage of vitamin D through our foods and in supplement form, but the best source is sunshine. Technically, vitamin D is not a vitamin. Vitamins are nutrients not produced by the body, so vitamin D is a steroid with hormone-like characteristics (Naeem, 2010). Being mindful of the risk of skin cancers due to overexposure to the sun, it's still important to have some daily interaction with the sun. Vitamin D deficiency is a global problem. It's estimated that 1 billion people worldwide (around 15%) lack this important vitamin, the situation declared a pandemic by WHO (Vitamin D Council, 2017), while one-third of all Australians are vitamin D deficient (Deakin University, 2012). Why is vitamin D so important to our health? It plays a significant role in the regulation of calcium and phosphorous levels in the blood – essential for healthy bones. The negative consequences of insufficient levels of this vital element are obesity, diabetes, hypertension, depression, fibromyalgia, chronic fatigue syndrome, osteoporosis, and neuro-degenerative diseases such as Alzheimer's disease. Some cancers such as prostate, breast and colon have been attributed to a lack of vitamin D. Heart disease, stroke, autoimmune diseases, birth defects, and periodontal disease can also be a consequence of a lack of vitamin D (Naeem, 2010). Am I frightening you? I hope not. I'm just trying to make you aware of how important this essential element is. You might ask if you are at risk of such a deficiency. If you have high levels of melanin in your skin, then your skin will be slow to produce the necessary levels of vitamin D. Similarly, if you block the ultraviolet B (UVB) rays with regular coats of sunblock, cover your skin with clothing, live and work indoors, are obese, elderly, or make a conscious decision to avoid the sun, then you're probably at risk of a deficiency (Naeem, 2010). Some of the symptoms that could suggest a vitamin D deficiency include becoming sick frequently especially with colds or the flu, regular infections, experiencing fatigue, bone and back pain, depression, slow wound healing, low bone density, and hair loss (Spritzler, 2016).

Before you strip off and run outside to bake in the sun, be mindful of the need for moderation. Professor Naeem (2010) advocates 15 to 20 minutes in the sunshine each day with a 40% skin exposure. However, there are important variables to consider when balancing our need for sun exposure with the risks associated with skin damage and skin cancer. While primarily focused on bone health, Osteoporosis Australia (2012) provides valid considerations on sun exposure, stating that it should be dependent on the season, our geographical location, what areas of skin are exposed, and skin types, cautioning us to have an awareness of these differences. For instance, in an Australian summer, mid-morning or mid-afternoon exposure is safer when ultraviolet (UV) radiation is likely to be lower. Cancer Council Australia (2016) has a position statement on the risks and benefits of sun exposure and vitamin D. They have an easy-to-read table outlining the average peak UV levels by month for each of the Australian capital cities. A useful rule of thumb is that sun protection is recommended once the UV index reaches 3 or above. There's a couple of ways you can determine the UV index: download the SunSmart app onto your iPhone, iPad or Android devices, or visit www.myuv.com.au. The day I visited the website, the reading was a maximum of 8.8 UV with sun protection recommended from 8.10 am to 3.00 pm for my location and the season.

You can also complement your vitamin D intake with food sources such as egg yolk, fatty fish (like canned tuna, mackerel, herring, or sardines), fortified dairy products, and beef liver (Naeem, 2010). There are supplement forms of the vitamin available and while these are reasonably adequate, they don't synthesise in the body as effectively as the real McCoy (MommyPotamus, 2018). So, for the good of your health and the many healthy years you'd like to be on this planet, just add a little sunlight to your health regime.

38. Slip, slop, slap

This alliterative triplet was the lynchpin for the Australian SunSmart campaign, the slogan and jingle first emerging back in 1981. Launched by Cancer Council Victoria, the promotion encouraged us to *slip* on a shirt, *slop* on the 30+ sunscreen and *slap* on a hat. The slogan now extends to *seeking shade or shelter and sliding on some sunnies.* The jingle is very much part of the Australian psyche and provides a powerful reminder to this day about the importance of reducing sun exposure and protecting ourselves against the increased risk of sun cancer. Australia's reputation as a sunburned country is true not only for the landscape, but its people. This wide brown land of ours has some pretty grim skin cancer statistics, despite the powerful campaign to protect us from the sun's harmful rays. According to Cancer Council Australia, two in three Australians will be diagnosed with skin cancer by the age of 70, with most forms of skin cancer being a direct result of sun exposure. Queensland, the state I hail from, has the highest rate of skin cancer in the world! I've had a couple of non-melanoma skin cancers removed myself: the legacy of sun exposure years earlier. It was a real wake-up call to take more care in protecting my skin when in the sun. Along with slopping on the sunscreen, I now wear a rash guard (rashie) – a lightweight, long-sleeved shirt made of spandex – when I'm out in the water. While it's not altogether attractive, I wear long-sleeved gloves when driving that I purchased through the Cancer Council. They protect my hands and arms from the sun as I'm driving, and I'm grateful for them. Cancer Council Australia reported that 13,314 Aussies were diagnosed with the most serious form of skin cancer – melanoma – in 2014 alone, with statistics also revealing that 2,162 Australians died as a result of some form of skin cancer in 2015 (Cancer Council Australia, 2018). There's been some recent research and development here in Australia around early detection of melanomas incorporating a world-first blood test designed to identify melanoma in its infancy. With this potentially deadly cancer claiming 1,500 lives each year, it's a vital step in reducing that mortality (Laurie, 2018). Whether you're an Australian reader or not, the importance of protecting your skin from overexposure to the sun cannot be overstated. Remember to *slip-slop-slap* so that you don't fall prey to this preventable but life-threatening condition.

39. Get grounded

Going barefoot is absolutely fabulous for your health. It is known as grounding, and in his publication *The Primal Connection* (2013), Mark Sisson argues that we've lost contact with the earth and its therapeutic electrical current since the arrival of footwear, housing, flooring, and elevated beds. Moreover, we are experiencing greater exposure to electromagnetic waves, Wi-Fi and mobile phones than ever before and with this exposure comes the potential for our enzyme function to be compromised (Pall, 2013, 2014).

So what's the connection between grounding and a healthy body? When you make a direct connection with the ground through walking, sitting or sleeping on the ground, you align with the earth's surface energy, allowing your body to return to its natural electrical balance. The beach or ocean is perhaps the best place to get grounded because the sand and water are highly conductive, and the water has high magnesium levels. (No wonder I sleep better when on a beach holiday!) As a consequence, Sisson suggests that the immune system is enhanced, allowing for a reduction in inflammation in our bodies.

There are said to be a myriad of other benefits too: reduction in chronic pain, higher energy levels, lower stress levels, the elimination of jet lag, relief from muscle tension and headaches, and the list goes on... One caution though folks: I'd be careful where you walk in bare feet: prickles, thorns and other unwelcome objects might catch you unawares. So check out your back garden, field or beach first for any potential hazards, then ditch your shoes and be one with the earth!

40. Get moving

By 'get moving', I'm not talking about taking off somewhere across the globe (however wonderful that might be). I'm referring to movement versus exercise. There's absolutely nothing wrong with exercise, but the real gifts in health come from simply moving your body. We're part of a generation that suffers from the sitting syndrome. How lethal this is to health was evidenced as far back as the 1950s when a study was undertaken comparing bus drivers (who sit) with their compatriots the bus conductors (who stand). The bus drivers were at twice the risk of developing heart disease. Our twenty-first century lifestyle has become a sitting time bomb.

According to Dr Michael Mosley (2015), the adverse effects of such a sedentary life include a 50% greater chance of developing type 2 diabetes and/or heart attack/stroke. Dr Mosley gives the sobering analogy that every hour spent watching television cuts 20 minutes off your life. Continuous sitting is a real problem, but there are very easy cures to counter this health crisis. Simply by standing and walking around every 30 minutes, you markedly reduce your blood sugar levels and insulin levels. If you've got a clever digital watch, it will tell you when it's time to stand at set intervals. It's so easy to become engrossed in what you're doing, lose track of time and forget to move. Dr Libby Weaver (2016a), one of my favourite nutritionists, suggests that a brisk 20-minute walk can help bowel movement for the constipated among us.

I found some great 'moving' tips from Shauna Mackenzie's Best Kept Self website. They are practical, fun and highly beneficial. Some of these include walking around while talking on the telephone or having a meeting; hanging from things (interesting!); squatting while reading a book (might be a little hard on the train though, so choose your spots thoughtfully); taking the stairs not the lift; and walking or biking rather than driving (Mackenzie, 2015). And as mentioned elsewhere in this book, gardening is a great form of movement – you get your vitamin D fix and some mobilisation of your joints through squatting.

In the brilliant film *The Big Fat Fix* (2016), there's a lot of discussion around the importance of moving your body, emphasising the greater flexibility, strength and balance of movement. Also, short, regular bursts of resistance training (rather than aerobic exercise) is another brilliant way to offset type 2 diabetes and metabolic syndrome through building insulin sensitivity, which allows the efficient utilisation of glucose. As expressed in the film, "movement heals: every time you move you floss your nerves...massage your organs...[and] circulate the blood".

Then there's the big public health message about 10,000 steps a day to keep you healthy. A Japanese researcher in the 1960s identified that most of us walked less than 4,000 steps a day. He found that by increasing them to 10,000, improved health was the result. This is a guideline for us to follow; 10,000 steps per day is a much healthier option than a sedentary lifestyle. However, a Scottish study on postal workers determined that the magic number is more likely 15,000 steps per day, with posties doing 15,000 steps more likely to have normal waistlines and no increased risk of diseases associated with a sedentary lifestyle (White, 2017). And by maintaining a walking pace of 5 kph (3 mph), you'll outwit and outpace the stalking pace of the grim reaper, according to a five-year Sydney study completed in 2011. The researchers analysed walking speed and mortality and drew on the fourteenth-century mythological and literary figure of the reaper as a comparison, who was said to walk at about 3 kph (1.8 mph). Rates of death were analysed and of the study's 1,705 male participants aged over 70, only those with a walking pace of 5 kph or more were able to maintain a safe distance from the grim reaper. In other words, keep moving at a brisk and steady pace to out-walk death (Stanaway *et al*, 2011).

We need only look to centenarian physician, Dr Shigeaki Hinohara, for evidence of these findings. He would take the stairs, rather than an elevator or escalator, two at a time, to get his muscles moving. He lived to be 105 years of age and worked until just a few months before his death (Gillett, 2017).

Now don't despair, once you make the decision to move, if you feel that the 15,000 steps mentioned earlier isn't achievable. However, if what I've already written doesn't inspire you, the following just might. I read in a newspaper the story of a young man who became an incomplete paraplegic after being hit by a truck. John Maclean became wheelchair-bound but with exercise-based treatments and resistance training, John discovered movement he didn't think was possible, as well as dramatically reducing his levels of pain. In a mere 17 months, he moved from paraplegic to able-bodied athlete, competing in a triathlon – a 1 km swim, 30 km bike ride and 10 km run (Gebilagin, *The Daily Telegraph*, 2017). So even when we think we've totally lost the ability, movement and resistance training can work wonders. Australia's oldest man at time of writing is 108 and he advocates a 45-minute "pretty rigorous" exercise regime each morning (Edmistone, 2017). Could this be the elixir of long life?

In sum, movement is medicine – it's free, and with none of the adverse side effects associated with medication.

41. Getting a good night's sleep

For some, getting a good night's sleep might be easy to achieve. But for others, it is the most yearned after and elusive of experiences. Matthew Walker (2017), author of *Why We Sleep* and director of the Center for Human Sleep Science at the University of California, says that sleep deprivation and fragmented sleep can have serious health implications. He suggests that among them are a greater risk of heart attack, obesity and stroke as well as a build-up of beta-amyloid, a toxic brain protein linked to Alzheimer's disease.

In her seminal work *From Exhausted to Energised* (2015), Dr Libby Weaver argues that good sleep is the basis of good health, yet statistically, more than half of us are unable to achieve this right to good health. If you have young children who require your attention during the night, only time and routine can 'remedy' this situation once the children grow and become more settled. However, do not despair: there are several important strategies you can employ to maximise healthy, natural sleep – and none of them involves taking sleeping tablets, counting sheep or wrestling with your pillow.

Weaver describes her approach as "sleep hygiene". She says that rest and sleep allow the kidneys to function well and that seven to nine hours of restorative sleep allow the kidneys to cleanse the blood, eliminating waste products in the urine the following morning (Weaver, 2013: 112). Firstly, if you're a caffeine drinker then make sure you have your caffeine hit(s) before midday. Caffeine can remain in your system for up to eight hours and keep you 'wired' and wakeful. You could try drinking water or herbal tea instead. Check in with yourself though: perhaps you're actually hungry, not thirsty, so keep some nuts handy as a snack.

Weaver's (2015) second strategy is to try some mindfulness or meditation before going to bed. Guided meditations are brilliant for relaxing the mind and body. As an addendum to this one, I've always found that before sleeping, I review my day and look for all the things I can be grateful for about those events. Inevitably, I fall asleep before I've completed my list and it's a wonderful way to slip into a dream state.

The next practical strategy for satisfying slumber is to keep your space clean and tidy and sleep between fresh sheets. It's hard to sleep in a messy environment. Also, washing your sheets regularly and allowing them to dry in the sun kills bacteria. It's a good idea to periodically air or vacuum mattresses where dust mites could reside: you don't want any nasty bed bugs!

Next, Weaver suggests avoiding backlit devices such as TVs, computers, iPads, iPhones, etc. about 90 minutes before going to bed. The electromagnetic field disrupts sleep patterns as well as depleting calcium in your body. If you really can't resist your smartphone or iPad before bed, then you do have another option. In a recent study in the *Journal of Psychiatric Research*, the wearing of amber-tinted lenses before sleep has been proven to block the blue light that interferes with sleep cycles, providing a further 30 minutes of sleep and reduced insomnia symptoms for the group studied (Shecter *et al,* 2018). When you eventually put the electronic gadgets to bed, Weaver (2015) suggests switching them to aeroplane mode. This eliminates those pesky notifications during the night, but you can still use your phone as an alarm to wake you in the morning.

Finally, here's a tip that I've learned from other sources over the years and it works really well for me. Try to make your bedroom as dark as possible, cutting out any light sources including LED lights from electrical gadgets. Artificial lights raise our cortisol levels, which disrupt sleep and are designed to wake you up. We've invested in roller blinds on the bedroom window to totally block any outside light and the 4.30 am sunrises in summer. When it's dark, our bodies pump out melatonin which regulates our sleep–wake cycle, lowering blood pressure, glucose levels and our body temperature – all the markers for great slumber. Hopefully, one or all of these tips will help you have a good and healthy night's sleep every night.

42. Breathing

What's the big deal with breathing? According to the experts, it's all about breathing *deeply* and from the *diaphragm*. When you effectively and routinely undertake deep breathing exercises, all manner of wonders occur. The oxygen you breathe in provides fuel for the vital organs – lungs, heart, liver, and kidneys. Mindful, deep breathing also improves brain function, aids the digestive tract, builds your immunity, lowers your blood pressure, restores your vitality, and is said to help deliver firmer, clearer skin, among so many other wonderful health benefits (Weaver, 2013: 154–158). Most of us use only about a third of our lung capacity, leaving stale and toxic air to circulate through our systems. (You just took a deep breath, didn't you? I did when I wrote this.)

Dr Libby Weaver (2013) writes earnestly about the importance of daily diaphragmatic breathing especially for alleviating stress, an aging and health-diminishing condition. Breathing is the only road to control our autonomic nervous system. Thinking our way to it won't work, as 'autonomic' implies that it's independent of the conscious mind. In other words, if you want a physiological shift to a calm state, the only way to do it is through breathing: it's crucial for promoting a calm state. And not only that, it shifts our chemistry from fat storage to fat burning.

According to Dr Jess Harvey (2014), a registered osteopath and advocate of Paul C Bragg's power breathing philosophy, the best way to maximise your lung capacity and thereby improve your health is to use your diaphragm. Harvey recommends that you breathe in using your tummy to expand forward, then breathe out, letting your tummy sink back in. For deeper cleansing, Harvey recommends pushing the diaphragm muscle down as you breathe in and pulling the tummy in and the diaphragm muscle up into the ribcage when you breathe out. If it sounds too complicated, simply start by taking 20 deep breaths periodically throughout the day or at a set time each day but persevere with the diaphragmatic breathing when you can. Perhaps you could do your deep breathing while the kettle boils for your cuppa each morning, or while you're having your morning shower. Whatever opportunity you decide on, make it a daily routine. But don't overdo it to the point of light-headedness, and especially not when driving or operating machinery!

43. Build muscle mass

If ever you were looking for a magic remedy for longevity, then building muscle mass through strength/resistance training has to come close. Forget those images of muscle-bound men and women posing in front of mirrors at their local gym, having just pressed or powerlifted X times their body weight for the perfect biceps, triceps, deltoids, pecs, and abs. That's bodybuilding and a whole other sphere outside of my experience and research (and capability if I'm honest). What I'm talking about is a little more modest, but it punches well above its weight in the longevity stakes. It's called resistance training and it's medicine for your body (Westcott, 2012).

In our 20s and 30s, we're probably at the pinnacle of physical strength, but after 30, our bodies naturally become physically weaker – unless we actively build muscle (Weaver, 2017). Studies have shown that the inactive among us lose between 3% and 8% of muscle mass per decade. On the flip side, the benefits of strength or resistance training are many and varied. Our physical performance is improved, and greater movement control is experienced. Our walking speed, functional independence, cognitive abilities, and self-esteem are all enhanced. The consequent reduction in visceral fat is said to prevent and manage type 2 diabetes, and cardiovascular health is enhanced due to a reduced blood pressure, lower LDL (bad) cholesterol levels and elevated HDL (good) cholesterol levels. Bone development may be promoted along with the possible reduction in back pain and the easing of the symptoms of arthritis and fibromyalgia (Westcott, 2012). And if you think that brawn and brains might be mutually exclusive, you will be pleasantly surprised to learn about a study that has found the stronger people become, the greater the benefit to their brain (The University of Sydney, 2016). The 'magic' I referred to earlier derives from the mitochondria. Our muscles contain the highest mitochondrial content of any tissue in the body. Building muscle mass reverses the loss of function in the mitochondria that occurs as we age. So, in effect, the aging process is halted at the level of our cells when we are doing exercise that builds muscle.

Before you dash out and buy yourself a gym membership or employ a personal trainer and start lifting weights, please know that strength training can be derived from a range of activities. Pilates provides great resistance training, while yoga uses your own body weight for the same purpose. Then, of course, there's a whole range of less formal activities such as gardening, walking, climbing stairs, and so on – all of which contribute to muscle building (Weaver, 2017). Whatever you choose to do to build muscle, know that undertaking at least two sessions per week and at high intensity will maximise the strength you gain (The University of Sydney, 2016). The bottom line is simple: the stronger you are, the longer you will live!

44. Dental hygiene

I've been visiting the dentist every year (sometimes twice per year) since I was a kid. Yeah, I know, I'm a dental nerd. However, I didn't always like dentist visits, especially if a cavity was detected and a filling required. Nonetheless, I learned early on (thanks to my parents for setting the dental trend) that taking care of my teeth was not just about dazzling others with a brilliant smile. While that might be important, dental care goes way beyond appearances; it's a foundation for good health.

According to the Queensland Government's Oral Health Unit (2017), oral hygiene in conjunction with appropriate dietary habits is essential for overall physical and emotional wellbeing. Bacteria that routinely live in your mouth can cause tooth decay and gum disease, leading to infections that often don't manifest symptoms until they've taken a real hold on your health. According to clinical trials, gum disease may also increase the risk of heart disease, diabetes, pneumonia, and premature birth (Rehme, 2005). I'm not going to scare you with too much gory detail, but my research revealed some fairly horrific dental stories that frightened the bejesus out of me. Suffice to say the dentist in question summed up by saying that dental infections, if left untreated, can eat through the skin on people's necks, choke off their airways, migrate to the heart, burrow into the brain, and... Okay, you get the picture and the message. Another brilliant way to inhibit these oral nasties is to floss daily. The *Journal of Aging Research* revealed the results of an oral health study of 5,611 older adults. The study compared those who brushed their teeth, flossed daily and made routine dentist visits with those who didn't follow this regime. Tooth brushing meant a 20–35% increase in longevity, while the flossers enjoyed a 30% increase in their lifespan over those who didn't floss (Paganini-Hill *et al*, 2011). The good news is that with regular brushing and flossing, plus a regular trip to your dentist, you'll be flashing those pearly whites with confidence knowing that you're dazzling on the inside and out.

45. Your GP: a portal to longevity

With the exception of families with children and those with ongoing ill-health, visiting your family doctor may well be something you only do when you absolutely have to and usually only when there's a health crisis. That's how I used to view my doctor visits. I took it as a 'badge of honour' when I hadn't been for a visit in a very long time. Not that there's anything wrong with my doctor. She's great: wise, patient, insightful. Now, through my research, I've come to appreciate the significant role that our general practitioners can make in our lives for maintaining that vim and vigour we're seeking, beyond the immediate response to ill-health and injury. It was a post-doctor visit that was part of the inspiration for this book.

The MacArthur Foundation, a philanthropic Chicago-based organisation that has established a research network into human longevity, identified three successful components to aging. Firstly, appropriate medical care. Secondly, ongoing physical and mental activity, and thirdly, an engagement in society (Second Opinion, 2016). These research findings seemed to privilege medical care over the other two options (discussed elsewhere here). Appropriate medical care is more about establishing a regular schedule of wellness appointments with your GP, alongside timely medical health visits for ill-health or injury. Developing an ongoing relationship with your doctor is an important way to manage your healthcare. In establishing this continued connection, your doctor will get to know you over time and become familiar with your medical history, which in turn fosters a trusting relationship. Dr Cody Dashiell of UCLA's David Geffen School of Medicine (2017) sagely commented that "discussing your care [with your doctor] when you are feeling well is the best way to prevent and treat illness in the future". The most common reason we attend our GP seems to be not for life-threatening or prevalent diseases but for less insidious conditions such as skin disorders like cysts, acne and dermatitis (Williams, 2013). While not diminishing the importance of these, our doctor is also the portal to significant preventative treatments for a host of potentially life-threatening illnesses. While the annual physical exam might be a little outdated, an annual visit to screen for specific areas of concern, potential risks and chronic conditions is an imperative. These include screening for breast, cervical, colorectal, and prostate cancers. While all these screenings are vital, I'll elaborate on colorectal cancer screening because colon cancer is the second most commonly diagnosed cancer in Australia, with symptoms rarely presenting themselves until the disease is advanced. The preparation for this test can be unpleasant (read 'yuck'), but it's preferable to prevent colon cancer than its alternative. If you have a family history, you are doing yourself a huge favour with early detection screenings. In 2017, statistics revealed that one in 13 Australians would be diagnosed with colorectal cancer by their eighty-fifth birthday. More immediately confronting is the estimated number of new cases for 2018, predicted to be 17,000, with 4,129 anticipated deaths among this number. On average, 80 Australians die from this disease each week. However, among all this gloom, the good news is that with early detection, 90% of cases are successfully treated (Cancer Australia, 2018).

Among the plethora of reasons you might need to visit your doctor, from acne to zygomycosis, the bottom line is the importance of making that wellness visit and having scheduled screenings as required. Your GP visit could mean the difference between living a long, independent, healthy, meaningful, enjoyable life because you've identified and dealt with any health challenges in a timely manner. Just one important viewpoint I'd like to add with regard to heeding your doctor's advice. This wisdom comes from Dr Shigeaki Hinohara, the Japanese doctor who studied longevity and lived to be 105 years old. Hinohara said that we should not blindly follow what our GP tells us but ask them if they would put their families through any of the procedures or surgeries they may be advocating for us. Doctors, like all of us, are human and don't have all the answers. Hinohara ministered to his patients with all the medical knowledge available to him but he was also a keen adherent of alternative therapies such as music or animal therapy as appropriate (Gillett, 2017).

46. Eye checks are health checks

I used to think that a yearly visit to the optometrist was all about checking whether my reading glasses needed an adjustment to the lens prescription, not whether my life depended upon it. I've since learned that there's so much more to this yearly visit to the eye doctor. If you're over 50, then I particularly encourage you to keep reading this topic, especially if a visit to an optometrist is not an annual calendar event. Once you hit your half century, your risk of having a range of serious eye diseases increases significantly. The story of Julie Beall might just be what you need to get you to that eye check-up (EyeMed, 2018). Julie's life ultimately hinged on what was discovered during her routine eye exam. Beall presumed that her deteriorating vision was related to fatigue and the need for reading glasses. Her eye examination revealed what the optometrist presumed was a detached retina. He was concerned and referred her to an ophthalmologist that same day. Beall was told she had choroidal melanoma, a potentially fatal form of cancer. Thankfully, this relatively early detection, quick responses from her eye specialists and a series of radioactive plaque therapy successfully treated Beall's eye disease. Eye examinations can also reveal other serious medical conditions such as high blood pressure, diabetes, elevated cholesterol, and heart disease (EyeMed, 2018). My Australian readers will be pleased to know that you receive Medicare benefits for eye examinations and the optometrist can even bill the government directly on your behalf (known as bulk billing), especially for children, pensioners and those with limited finances (Optometry Australia, 2018). My understanding is that most Americans receive benefits through their employer, but that the original Medicare and the Affordable Care Act don't cover regular adult vision checks (EyeMed, 2018).

You can also protect your eyes from damage by wearing a good pair of UV protective sunglasses. Optometry Australia (2018a) says that donning such sunglasses during the daylight hours protects eyes from the sun's harmful ultraviolet rays, which could otherwise lead to cataracts. They also protect against the blue light from the solar spectrum that might increase your risk of macular degeneration. And from a purely aesthetic perspective, you'll be guarding against premature wrinkling around your eyes. It's often been said that the eyes are a window into the soul: I believe they're a window into the health of your body too.

47. Yoga

It's probably no surprise that this form of mind and body exercise should be included as one of the important 100 activities or actions for healthy longevity. My mother was an early participant in the practice of yoga and she introduced me to it when I was about 16. (My mum's now 85 and living independently with relatively good health, so I'd like to think that her early yoga may have supported her.) Back in the day, I'd don a black jumpsuit, grab a towel and accompany her to a neighbour's home where we stretched and twisted and breathed our way to a Zen state. Well, maybe not quite *that* chilled, but as I was a relatively anxious individual, it was indeed very emotionally rewarding, and physically gratifying too. Yoga combines mindfulness and movement, helping you to breathe through any stress and relax and soothe the muscles. Of course, when I started yoga back in the 1970s, there was only one form of it that I was aware of. Nowadays there's hatha, vinyasa, Iyengar, Ashtanga, Bikram, hot yoga, Kundalini, yin yoga, doga (yoga with dogs!) and more, half of which I cannot even pronounce! The Gaiam website provides a brief explanation of the various forms of yoga if you're interested (Gaiam, 2016). If you're new to yoga, then it would probably be best to start with a general form such as hatha, a generic term for any yoga that provides a gentle introduction to the basic physical postures.

Now for the benefits, and I can tell you there are many! I'll mention just a few I consider to be 'sexy' and provide you a reference to the rest. For starters, you'll find that you will sleep better and generally feel happier due to increased serotonin levels. A sharper focus is another benefit that translates to improved coordination, reaction time and memory, and an enhanced IQ. Yoga practice has been known to benefit your relationships: with its emphasis on avoiding harm to others, speaking your truth, and taking only what you need, these are all-important elements towards strong foundations in a relationship.

Timothy McCall (2007) outlines other benefits of practising yoga regularly. And don't feel you have to join a class, especially if the tyranny of distance or other circumstances prevent you from getting to a regular class. There are loads of great DVDs as well as online material. In one of her regular online posts, Dr Libby Weaver says that yoga and Pilates are brilliant for gut function. They strengthen core muscles that in turn support the efficient elimination of waste products from our bodies (Weaver, 2016a). With that said, all you really need is some space to stretch, a mat or towel, comfortable clothing, and an open mind to the benefits of this modality. You'll probably be moving from child's pose to handstand in no time, lengthening your body and the years on this planet too!

48. Get on ya bike

It's been proven that when you get on your bike and undertake high-intensity interval training (HIIT), you are cycling your way to a younger, healthier you. The theory is that these HIIT short-burst exercise programs, coupled with brief recovery periods of low-intensity training, rejuvenate the body's 'batteries', the body's mitochondria that provide our energy. As we age (even from our 20s), their 'charge' declines, and it does so *rapidly* for the elders among us.

Findings in a 2017 US study published in *Cell Metabolism* revealed that HIIT actually reverses the loss of function in the mitochondria which, in effect, halts the aging process at the level of our cells. The fuel from the nutrients we eat is converted into energy-carrying molecules essential for all cellular processes. A pretty impressive and important function! The study was conducted over 12 weeks and involved subjects aged 18–30 and 65–80 years of age. All volunteers undertook three different modalities – HIIT, resistance training and combination training. HIIT was a hit. It provided the most pronounced benefits, especially among the older age group: their mitochondrial function increased by around 69% compared to the younger subjects with a 49% improvement (Robinson *et al*, 2017).

And there's benefits to your immune system as well. A University of Birmingham study in 2018 compared active adult cyclists aged 55–79

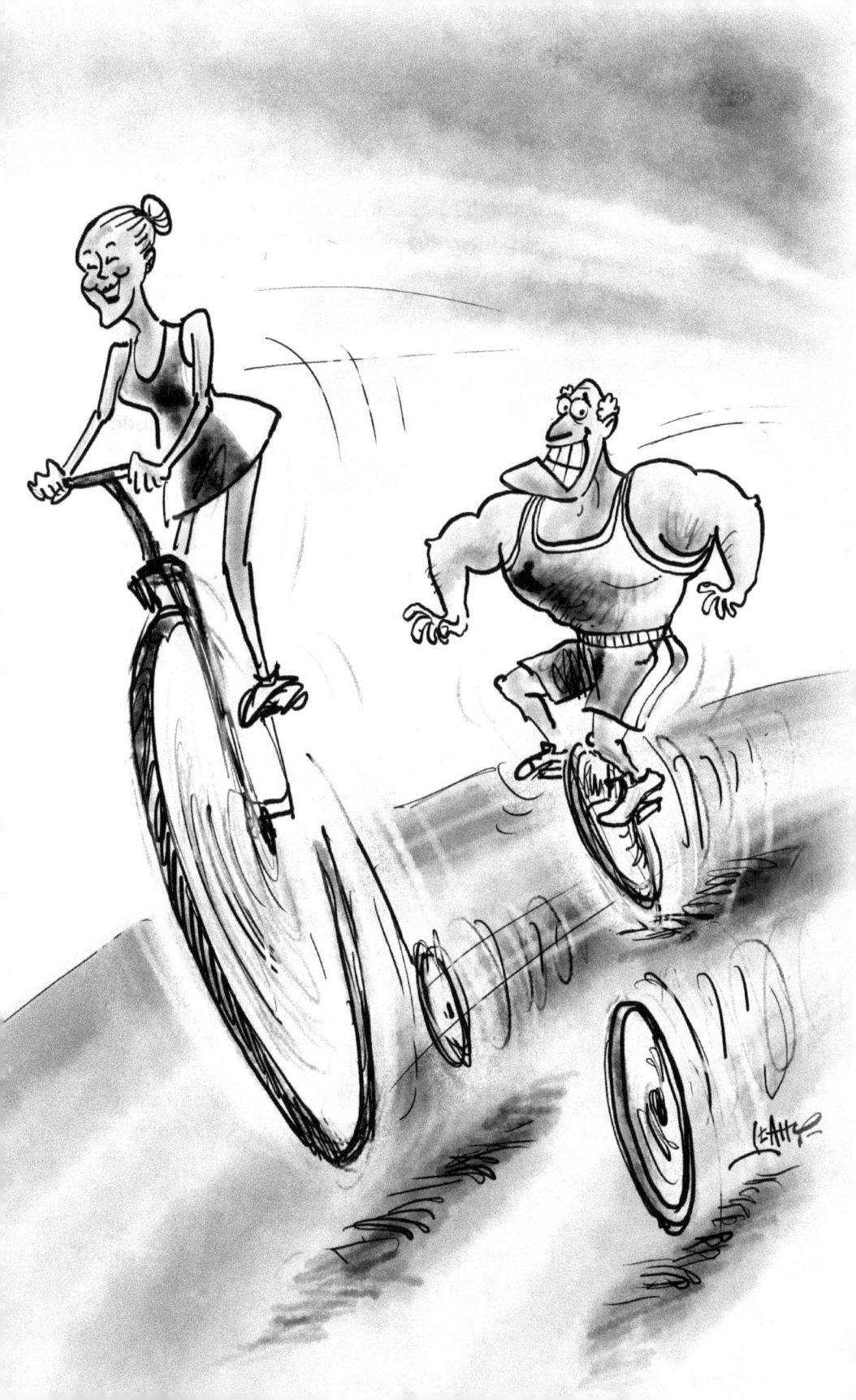

with their less-than-active counterparts, along with adults aged 20–36. The study showed that the T-cells in the older active cyclists were much higher than in the non-active subjects, and they were at the same level as the younger cohort. The older active cyclists had the immune systems of 20-year-olds. What it all comes down to is that a stronger immune system makes you less susceptible to infections, rheumatoid arthritis and potentially, cancer (Sifferlin, 2018). In applying the HIIT approach to cycling, it's important to take note of its short-burst-then-low-intensity-recovery nature, as opposed to the training you might do for, say, the Tour de France. Professional cyclists are said to have a life expectancy 15 years *lower* than the average population primarily because of the endurance nature of their physical routines. They are more likely to develop 'athletic heart' (enlarged heart), which makes them more susceptible to sudden cardiac arrest (Xtend Life, 2011).

There's a bicycling specialist website that outlines HIIT cycling sessions (Yeager, 2018). They propose twice-weekly sessions known as 'Quick 'n Dirty 30s'. Thirty seconds is believed to be the ultimate HIIT duration. Warm up for 10 minutes then push as hard as you can for 30 seconds, pedal easy for 60 seconds (90 for beginner cyclists), repeat four times, then pedal easy for four minutes. You can repeat the sequence twice more and then cool down for five minutes. There's also a focused fat-burning HIIT session on this website for the ultimate enthusiast (Yeager, 2018).

Whether it's an exercise bike, indoor static bike trainer in your garage or gym or the two-wheeler you're scooting around the suburbs on, give yourself permission to do a 30-minute HIIT workout, knowing that you're probably adding a few more good years to your life. Remember not to push yourself beyond your ability and if you're able to, get guidance from a recommended personal trainer or gym instructor. If you needed further convincing on the merits of cycling, then you need look no further than French supercentenarian, Jeanne Calment, who died in 1997 at the lovely old age of 122. One of her secrets (despite a steady diet of chocolate and port) was riding her bike until she was 100 (McKay, 2017).

49. Swim for your life

I've talked about various forms of exercise elsewhere in this book, but hands down in my experience, regular swimming is the best and safest form of exercise regardless of age or fitness level. It's marvellous for your emotional and mental wellbeing and is relatively inexpensive and accessible for those who live near swimming lanes or a safe watercourse. Here in Australia, most of the population clings to the coastline like frogs around a pond, dotted along the eastern, southern and western seaboards of this vast continent. While ocean swimming is restricted or cautioned in some parts of the country due to hazardous marine life and other factors, lap pools are a feature of many urban and regional areas. And there's always the backyard swimming pool for those fortunate enough to have one, which can be equipped with a stationary harness to provide endless hours of 'lap' swimming.

The health benefits of swimming are almost unparalleled by any other sport. American fitness legend, Jack LaLanne, is testament to the health and longevity benefits of swimming. He lived to the ripe old age of 94 and incorporated swimming as an important part of his fitness regime. This is backed up by a study conducted by the Counsilman Center for the Science of Swimming Human Performance Laboratory at Indiana University. They determined that regardless of age, swimmers had a lower risk of developing cardiovascular disease (Hardesty, 2017). Here are just some of the benefits of a consistent swimming program: core strength and stability are improved; aerobic fitness is improved; HDL (the good cholesterol) is enhanced; you'll experience a decrease in triglycerides (a type of fat found in the blood); blood pressure will lower along with a reduction in total cholesterol; and there's improvement in strength, muscle tone and power. On top of all that, if you have orthopaedic issues such as back or knee problems, the buoyancy of the water will reduce the impact on your body, thus alleviating pain while improving your range of motion. It's also a valuable form of exercise for those wanting to lose weight, and when coupled with a healthy eating plan, you'll look trim, taut and terrific in no time. Additionally, swimming's a great stress management tool. The water can be a soothing and calming environment that can leave you feeling in a meditative state (Hardesty, 2017).

I'd like to add another benefit from personal experience. I started swimming training about four years ago, joining an adult squad at my local pool. Admittedly I'm no fish, and tend to swim in the slow swimmers' lane, but I've discovered the wonderful camaraderie and social banter that goes along with our training. We've got a brilliant swim coach, Phil, who tailors our training to our ability. Phil tells the best bad Dad jokes to break up the session a little and keep the momentum going, so we have a few laughs and I've made some close friends as well. Social connection is important, as it's proven to be a crucial ingredient for a long life. Perhaps it's time to dig that swimsuit out from the bottom drawer, don a cap and goggles and get into the pool. Oh, and if you're swimming in open water, please stay safe, be aware of currents and any other dangers, and have a swimming buddy along to enjoy the experience.

50. Dance your way to good health

I've chatted elsewhere about the benefits of spontaneity, joy and uninhibited actions such as taking a skip down the aisle of your shopping centre to add years to your life (see the section *Don't act your age – act younger*), but there's also dance – regular and consistent – to help you sidestep the aging process physically, mentally and emotionally.

Medical practitioner Richard Baxter's speciality area is plastic surgery, but he's discovered a number of wonderful benefits to dancing for retaining our youth, all without the use of a scalpel or Botox syringe. It does, however, require you to strap on your dancing shoes. Canadian researchers from the International Laboratory for Brain, Music and Sound Research at McGill University in Montreal have found that long-term dance training improves the grey and white matter of the brain (Baxter, 2014). Grey matter is the grey nerve cell bodies; white matter are the nerve fibres. This is known as 'brain plasticity'. Dancing allows for a rewiring of the brain, preserving cognitive function as we age. It's probably no surprise to learn that dancing also helps maintain balance. For those who have experienced illnesses that have affected physical and mental functioning, it's an excellent rehabilitation tool, addressing not only the physical and motor skill requirements, but also cognitive functions such as perception, emotion and memory. Researchers Dhami, Moreno & DeSouza (2015) echo Baxter's work in this area, noting the enjoyment factor as a means of healing through the interactive nature of dance (Dhami, Moreno & DeSouza, 2015). As Baxter notes, the joy that can derive from dance is said to lessen depression. A group of elderly nursing home residents reduced their anti-depression medications following weekly dance classes! It's also been proven that you develop improved muscle mass for strength and endurance and enhance your cardiovascular health. Baxter followed studies from Trent University in Nottingham in the United Kingdom that found dance provides a natural high. Dancers report mood enhancement, socialising and escapism as motivators for their continued engagement (in Baxter, 2014). What a healthy way to experience a sense of euphoria when compared to riskier alternatives such as gambling, drinking or drug-taking.

While this next benefit of dance has not been scientifically proven, it does have a cause and effect relationship. A cardiac research team in Brazil speculated that sexual function could be enhanced because dance styles such as salsa, merengue and samba often induce the 'happy hormones' – endorphins. It's all got to do with the combination of physical activity and music in these dance forms. Of all the fitness training you might choose to adopt for health and wellbeing, apparently none compares with dancing for reversing the signs of aging (Rehfeld *et al*, 2017). Whether it's the Argentine tango, the paso doble or square dancing, there's one thing for sure: dance has a huge potential for slowing down and reversing the aging process.

51. Happy, healthy feet: a step in the right direction

I recently read an article *Happy Feet* (Bee, 2018), discussing the lack of focus we give to this most important part of our bodies, and how imperative good foot health is to our overall wellbeing. I have to be honest that I haven't always taken an interest in my feet, nor given them the care they deserve until injury, strain, aches, and pains have forced me to glance in their direction. Yet they have helped me skip, trudge, run, gallop, plod, tiptoe, scamper, sidestep, and scurry my way through the world, without a second thought most of the time. I've squeezed them into stilettos, wrangled them into a range of runners, gym shoes and exercise boots, all in the hope of putting my best foot forward – to impress someone, to pound the pavement for umpteen kilometres to the gods of fitness or simply to get from A to B. With this sort of neglect, we'll eventually foot the bill in bouts of pain, fallen arches or the need for medical attention of some kind.

The importance of caring for our feet is an ancient modality. Carvings dating back to 2400BC in the Egyptian tomb of a royal physician depict care of the feet and hands in bas relief (Snodgrass, 2013), and Hippocrates practised an early form of reflexology to rid the body of 'residues' (Basis, 2018). Our feet are a good barometer for the early warning signs of life-threatening conditions. Any changes to the skin, nails or sensation could be a sign of something wrong with our overall health. Podiatrist Carolyn McAloon tells us that because our feet are furthest from our heart and spine they're the first indicator of nerve damage issues. Our bodies, in their infinite wisdom, will send blood supply to vital organs and the brain before sending any to our extremities when we experience a health crisis, so while that's not good for our feet, they will give us signs and symptoms to alert us to serious health issues and the need to act. In this regard, they are lifesavers (Elias, 2013). Foot cramps, for example, could be a sign of serious circulation or nerve issues, or a relatively harmless signal of a mineral deficiency (magnesium, for instance), or the need to drink more water because we're dehydrated. More seriously, persistently sore heels can be a red flag for diabetes, or planta fasciitis, a painful condition where the thick, supportive band of tissue that runs along the bottom of the foot to the heel becomes strained. Getting cold feet is a non-life-threatening condition if we're feeling anxious about a momentous event, but not if it might suggest hypothyroidism: an inability to warm the feet. A thyroid problem can be associated with hair loss, extreme tiredness, weight gain, and depression. Other conditions of the feet include flakiness, itchiness, peeling, and excessive sweat. With all these foot challenges to consider, it makes absolute sense that we should take notice of, care for and appreciate these important extremities, especially if they give us signs and symptoms of potentially life-threatening ailments. Take notice of your feet and be aware of any changes or discomforts, as these could be indicators of deficiencies or illness elsewhere in your body. Allowing yourself some barefoot time is good foot therapy, as I've outlined under the topic *Get grounded*.

Soaking your feet in a solution of warm water and salt or magnesium is ideal for cramps and stressed feet. An important element to this soak is to include a simple but effective move called foot 'doming' whereby you use the foot muscles to create a dome by pulling the toes towards your nose, elevating the arch. It'll strengthen and lengthen the muscles in your foot (Bee, 2018). This is a good ongoing maintenance exercise for strengthening your foot muscles. Another involves removing your socks and simply wriggling your toes, then trying to pick up something like marbles. You can also practise writing the alphabet with your toes or grabbing a towel with your feet for foot core stability. Training your muscles in this way is similar to the core exercises you might do for your abdomen. Stronger foot muscles lead to better posture and a reduction in back pain, as your feet provide a more stable foundation.

I mentioned reflexology earlier associated with our ancient friend, Hippocrates. It's a popular modality today, the principle being that there are nerve endings in our hands and feet that correspond to muscles and organs in our body. By applying pressure to points in the hands and feet, this reflexology process is said to relax tension, improve circulation and promote general health (Bauer, 2015). So why don't you have a foot in both camps – an awareness of and a care for your feet, as a way of ensuring you've got happy feet. And you might just reduce the risk of having one foot in an early grave, at least not before your hundredth-plus birthday!

52. Get a spinal adjustment

Some years ago, I was suffering from severe neck spasms as a result of an old injury, aggravated by hours of computer work. The pain was so debilitating that I could barely move, let alone drive anywhere to get help. The nearest medical aid was a chiropractor who had recently set up his practice in the village shopping complex three minutes from our home. I wasn't averse to alternative therapies and any healing hands were welcome in that moment. I asked my friend and neighbour if she'd drive me there. The short journey was excruciating and seemed interminable, not because of my friend's driving (she drove with care and I was grateful to her), but because every little bump, turn and wrinkle in the road aggravated the spasms. Thankfully, the waiting room was quiet when we arrived, so I managed to get in for an appointment almost immediately. The chiropractor was a big man, at least six foot five, and I noticed, as I took in the enormity of his frame, that he had hands the size of dustbin lids (I'm almost not joking)! I was to learn from subsequent appointments that he was a former All Blacks rugby union player from New Zealand who'd settled in Australia with his family after retiring from the game.

Despite his intimidating size and those hands, he proved to be a gentle giant, and very practised and thorough in his art. He immediately provided some relief with gentle adjustment, and insisted on x-rays to eliminate the possibility of anything more sinister. My recovery was swift, and I was back slogging away at the keyboard in no time. This extraordinary practitioner became our family chiro for many years until his eventual return to his native New Zealand. Anyone who's ever experienced extreme pain followed by magical and immediate relief will understand my deep gratitude and appreciation for those who provide that deliverance. If I have a bias in favour of chiropractic adjustments, then I blame this wonderful practitioner. Suffice to say, I've managed to convince my partner of its merits and we're just about chiropractic junkies, with monthly maintenance checks. They've proven to be an essential element to our musculoskeletal health and overall wellbeing.

The term 'chiropractic' derives from the Greek *cheir* (hand) and *praxis* (practice), suggesting hands-on therapy. It was founded by Daniel David Palmer in the United States in 1895. Chiropractic adopts a similar philosophy to healing as in Eastern medical practices. It's based on the concept of vitalism, contrasting with the mechanist approach in Western medicine. Each has its place in healing the body. As the name implies, a mechanist approach to healing views the body as various mechanical systems, each system requiring separate and specialist care either through medications or perhaps surgery. Vitalism assumes that there is an innate intelligence and order within the body that is designed to heal us, and that all the body's systems are interconnected rather than isolated. When the vertebrae experience an interruption (otherwise known as a subluxation), the body's ability to heal itself is disrupted. Conversely, when a subluxation is corrected with gentle and precise adjustments, this innate intelligence helps the body to function at optimum health. In many ways, the chiropractor is the conduit for the body to do its own healing. Alongside this innate wisdom, the chiropractor brings precision and knowledge to working with their patients for healing to occur (Wilderness Chiropractic, 2012). I didn't know any of this when I gingerly hobbled into my first chiropractic appointment all those years ago, but it makes sense that well aligned vertebrae support our musculoskeletal system for enhanced health.

A range of research has established that musculoskeletal adjustments via a chiropractor result in improvement in neck pain, shoulder and neck trigger pain and sports injuries (Salehi, 2015). While this study of a range of research papers could not confirm benefits beyond these areas, it has been argued that the modality has even broader health benefits. Chiropractic adjustments are said to alleviate asthma symptoms, infant colic, autism spectrum disorder, gastrointestinal problems, fibromyalgia, back pain, and carpal tunnel syndrome. And with the intrinsic association between the nervous system and the brain in chiropractic, these adjustments are said to improve mental health as well as enhance sleep, increase energy levels and improve posture (Pain Doctor, 2016). The nervous system coordinates the spine and the musculoskeletal system and as such is imperative to our health and wellbeing. If these gentle and precise adjustments can support that system, guided by a wise practitioner, then it's an adjustment to your health that might be worth considering.

53. Massage your way to good health

While the main reason many of us have a massage is to relax, you might be surprised at the abundance of other health benefits that a good massage can bring. As a generation of 'sitters', our posture is overloaded, leading to postural stress manifesting as lower back pain and tight gluteal muscles. Massage can counteract this imbalance by loosening and stretching the tight muscles. In a 2011 study in the *Annals of Internal Medicine*, it was found that massage therapy was just as effective as other methods for treating chronic back pain (Cherkin *et al*, 2011). Massage also increases and improves circulation. Moreover, it soothes anxiety and depression. Human touch that is safe, professional and friendly is said to be therapeutic and relaxing, so says Canadian registered massage therapist and kinesiologist, Katharine Watts (Watts, 2017). We often hear that stress can be a killer, so if massage reduces stress it's got my tick of approval for realising healthy longevity. Massage is also said to improve sleep, the more relaxed state allowing you to drift into dream world without having to count all those pesky sheep.

But wait, there's more: your immune system is also boosted because the white blood cell count is increased, thus playing a role in fending off disease. The Buck Institute for Research on Aging in the US takes this further, finding that having a 10-minute massage following exercise promoted the growth of new mitochondria. Mitochondria is the cell 'control centre'. Some sources argue that there are about 10 million billion of them in the body and their job is to use the oxygen we breathe to power our bodies. When the mitochondria is in decline, so are we: it's called aging (Foster, 2018)! If a 10-minute massage can help reverse the aging process, bring it on! And if headaches are your problem, especially when associated with tension, then a massage might just be the modality for you in preference to paracetamol.

A Northumbria University study of couples undergoing a three-week massage course revealed that recipient and masseur were equally rewarded, both reporting reduced stress. Sayuri Naruse, the lead author of the study, argues that massage can be an effective way for couples to improve physical and emotional wellbeing, with the added benefit of showing affection to each other (Whiteman, 2017).

54. Dry body brushing

Body brushing is based on Ayurvedic medicine and is designed to stimulate your skin, encouraging a shift in the circulation from the internal to the external vessels and promoting the lymphatic system to drain its collected fluid. Unlike the heart, the lymphatic system doesn't have a pump, so it relies on either movement or massage to shift any stagnant flow. It's best to use a brush with natural fibres that are firm yet gentle on your skin, with a long handle for those hard-to-reach places like the middle of your back. Use circular strokes and a gentle pressure: you don't want to scratch your skin!

The dry brushing technique also gently removes dead skin cells, leaving the skin soft, supple and refreshed. Some of the other benefits of dry body brushing include enhancing your immunity, improving skin health and appearance, better blood circulation which stimulates the removal of waste products, and a reduction in cellulite. The exfoliation of old skin cells will leave you feeling revitalised. Ideally, it's best to dry body brush before showering in the mornings: that way you can rinse away any impurities and start the day with a glow. Once a week is probably frequently enough, as brushing too often may break down the skin's protective barriers. A note of caution: if you have sensitive skin or you develop a sensitivity to dry body brushing, it's best to cease the practice. If you're new to it, test a patch of your skin a few times first – either on your arm or your leg (Healthy Home Economist, 2018).

55. Long life is just a s-t-r-e-t-c-h away

I've alluded to the importance of stretching in several other areas of the book, in particular with regard to yoga and massage. However, in researching this book, I've come to recognise the important association between stretching and a healthy long life, so I feel it's worthy of its own discussion. Oh, and did I mention that it'll make you look younger too? More of that in a moment. We've moved into a 'stretch revolution', with advocates claiming there are more benefits to developing our flexibility through stretching than there are through workouts. Such is the enthusiasm for this form of exercise that there are now dedicated 'stretch studios' where you pay anything from $39 to $100 a session for assisted stretching. But as Holly Brasher of the Australian Physiotherapy Association says, while being assisted to stretch has proven to increase your range and muscle flexibility and perhaps also keep you more accountable, it's somewhat of a luxury which can, with discipline and direction, be done on your own (Mayoh, 2018). Irrespective of whether you're stretching solo, in a group or assisted, the health benefits are enormous. For starters, you'll reduce your muscle tension, increase the range of movement in your joints and improve muscle coordination. On top of all that, you'll increase your blood circulation which leads to greater energy levels (Cosman, 2017). Just as significantly, stretching helps us look younger, the theory being that releasing the fascia that surrounds our muscles makes us look more youthful. Fascia is akin to a web or net that scaffolds our muscles. When we're young, the fibres in fascia are neat and have symmetry but as we age, these become tangled. As we stretch our muscles, the fascias in our lower limbs that can pull on our face are released, leaving us with a more lifted and youthful glow (Wylde, 2017). While this might be stretching things a little and drawing a long bow between smooth fascia and smooth facial skin, it's certainly worth trying, just in case. Other positive results of stretching are that you'll lift your mood with the resultant endorphin release, lower your LDL (bad) cholesterol and raise your HDL (good) cholesterol levels, improve your flexibility, lessening the likelihood of injury during activities, and improve your posture through enhanced spinal alignment (Cosman, 2017).

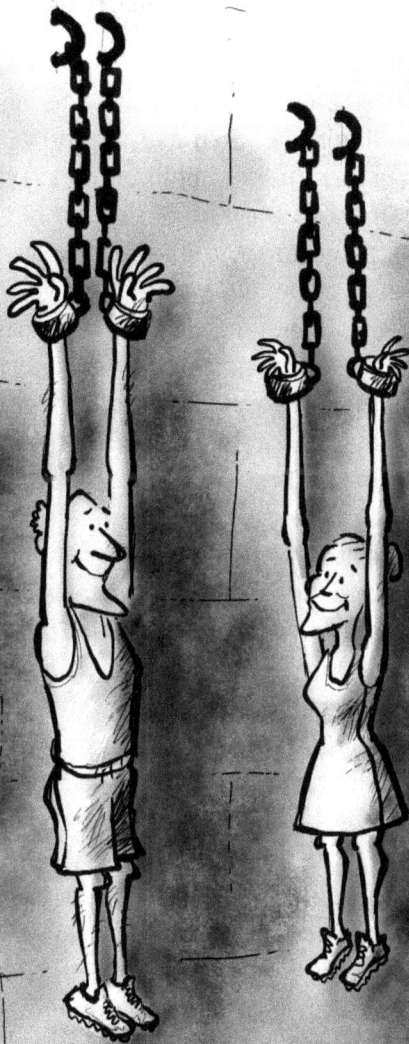

I'll outline several stretches, although one in particular is paramount to our wellbeing. Known as the hip flexor, this primary muscle attaches your femur or thigh bone to your pelvis and lumbar spine. Its main function is to assist the hip joints to move properly through their full range. It enables you to draw your legs to your torso, as well as allowing you to pivot your legs from side to side and backwards. It's the muscle that stabilises your hips and lower body, maintaining strength in your pelvis and lumbar spine. Being the connecting muscle for your torso and legs, the hip flexor allows your legs to move in combination with your torso. In short, just as the ancient Romans bragged that 'all roads lead to Rome', when it comes to stretching, everything is connected through your hips! As fitness author and personal trainer Mike Westerdal says, tight or locked hip flexors are often associated with joint, leg and back pain, walking with discomfort, hips locking up, poor posture, sleeplessness, low energy, and high anxiety (Westerdal, 2018). No matter your age or activity level, if the hip flexors are not kept stretched and in good condition, many a common health (and sometimes chronic) condition emerges as a result of neglect or lack of awareness.

So let's look at how to stretch the hip flexor as well as some other all-important stretches. Sports medicine physiotherapist Catherine Potter (2013) says that you should stretch daily. Before stretching, Potter cautions you to warm up (e.g. by running on the spot, or taking a brisk walk, until you develop a mild sweat). She also says that the stretches need to be done in a slow and controlled way with no bouncing, and that if any pain is experienced, to cease the stretch immediately. Westerdal recommends the hip flexor stretch first thing in the morning. He calls it the '90 90 kneeling stretch with side bending'. Sounds complicated but it's not. I would explain this hip flexor stretch here for you, but as a picture paints a thousand words, Westerdal's short YouTube clip demonstrates the hip flexor well (see my *Reference List* at the back of this book). While you're probably unfamiliar with the hip flexor stretch, it is a vital one for overall good health.

It's also a good idea to include in your daily routine the stretches you are more familiar with. There are several ways to do a hamstring stretch, but this one seems the most popular.

1. Stand with the leg to be stretched a little in front of the other.
2. Bend the back knee.
3. Lean forward from the hips.
4. Place your hand on the bent leg's thigh for balance. You can lean further forward if you don't feel a stretch.

Next is your gluteus maximus (aka 'glute' or 'butt muscle').

1. Lie on your back.
2. Using your hands, take your knee to your opposite knee until you feel a stretch in your buttocks or the front of your hips.
3. Hold for 10–30 seconds and repeat four times for a moderate stretch.
4. Repeat on your other side.

The quadriceps stretch is also a goodie but take it easy if you're prone to knee or lower back pain. For a standing quad stretch:

1. Reach back and grab your left foot in your left hand, keeping your thighs aligned and your left leg in line with the hip.
2. Breathe deeply and hold for 10–30 seconds.
3. Repeat on the other side.

For a chest stretch:

1. Stand in the middle of a doorway, one foot in front of the other.
2. Bend your elbows to a 90° angle.
3. Place your forearms on each side of the doorway, shifting your weight onto your front leg, then lean forward until you feel a stretch in your chest muscles (Potter, 2013).

I recommend watching Potter's video (see *Reference List* for web link) for a more comprehensive range of stretches and to get the advantage of the visual demonstrations.

And remember, this section is a general guide only to stretching and doesn't replace the advice you should receive from a qualified health professional before beginning any new exercise regime. Once you've been given the all-clear, I suggest you start your stretching program gradually. It may take several weeks to see significant results, but be patient and persistent with this most important element for a longer, healthier and more youthful you.

56. Roll your way to good health

Once upon a time the foam roller was synonymous with elite athletes who released their taut muscles in a process known as 'self-myofascial release' (SMR) (Rodie, 2017; Myers, 2015). Sounds like a form of torture or self-flagellation, doesn't it! But rolling has become a very popular and effective pastime among the elite and non-elite among us. Today, these rollers are readily available from department stores and health practitioners. Where once you would have to spend money on physiotherapists, massage therapists and other 'ists' and 'paths' to sort out your knots and tight spots, you've now got this do-it-yourself tool. I first spotted a compressed foam roller in my osteopath's practice and as a curious being, enquired about its uses and benefits. So impressed was I that I bought one, armed with clear instructions from my osteopath. I have discussed earlier about how stretch smooths out the fascia (the webbing that surrounds our muscles) but a good rolling also encompasses the nerve cells, muscle and epithelia (membranous tissue covering the internal organs). Physiotherapist Scott Wilson (in Rodie, 2017) says that regular rolling reduces inflammation, scar tissue and joint stress, while also improving circulation and flexibility. He says that rolling can improve your posture and aid in better sleep. Tom Myers (2015) is a specialist in the area of SMR, so I'm drawing on his wisdom primarily in relaying the importance and the how-to of foam rolling.

The need to release the congestion that builds up in our muscles was recognised by the famous sixteenth-century physician Paracelsus, who wrote. "There is one disease, and its name is congestion." Relieving and clearing the congestion of the muscles is what rolling is all about. To put it another way, "Water still: poison. Water moving: life" (Bedouin proverb). Myers draws an analogy between a sponge full of water and the epithelial and muscle tissues. He says that when rolling we are squeezing the water from these tissues and they are sucked back in again as we release the roller, just as we squeeze a sponge over the sink and then let the water refill it when washing the dishes. This releasing and replenishing process is a good thing because, among other things, it hydrates the area. While it may not make our muscles stronger, Myers argues there is evidence to suggest that it does make our arteries more elastic. Rolling can be a painful process especially if, like me, you've never rolled or had much massaging of tight muscles. However, as Myers maintains, if it's 'sensationful' (i.e. painful) and causes muscle contraction and cellular reaction, that's a negative. He argues that it's preferable to stay in the pleasurable realm or the 'hedonic point' between pleasure and pain. Nevertheless, if the area hurts, it does mean it needs your attention. Focusing on the area on the border of the painful spot is a good place to start.

There are three key points to SMR through rolling that yield the best results. Firstly, move slowly, as this allows for deeper release of tissue, as opposed to fast rolling which can result in bruising, muscle tension and sensory receptor damage. Secondly, look for the hidden tight spots. By continually rolling the same areas you'll diminish the efficacy of rolling. Rather, roll different parts of your body such as the upper part of the inner thigh (if you can manage it), the front and back of your armpit, or manipulate the roller to reach different parts of your back. The third key point to rolling is to hold the roller still. As you move over the roller you are breaking up the adhesions between fascial planes (Myers, 2015). Having said all this, you can begin with the four main areas: upper back, iliotibial band (ITB) – a band of muscle that runs laterally along the thigh from the pelvis to the tibia, the gluteus medius – the mid-section of your butt, and the calves. Personal trainer Lauren Roxburgh (in Rodie, 2017) says that the foam roller is a "workout and stability apparatus...that can decrease stress, increase body awareness, gain streamlined definition, a new glow and a calmer vibe" (Rodie, 2017). Recently, I've found rollers online for $24 including delivery in Australia, so they're relatively inexpensive for the benefits derived. The most important take-home message about rolling is to do it mindfully, slowly and perceptively in a way that addresses the tight areas of your body without being painful.

57. Mud up

If you were ever a fan of the television series *Suits*, you're probably visualising the character Louis Litt neck deep in a bath of mud. This tip doesn't ask that much of you, although a full immersion in a mud bath is likely to be a wonderful spa experience. My mud is the bentonite clay kind, also known as montmorillonite clay, named after the French region where the clay was first discovered. It's a healing clay used both internally and externally. Derived from the ash of volcanoes, it has been used therapeutically for centuries for those seeking to detoxify their bodies and as a defence against illnesses (Wellness Mama, 2017). I first encountered the clay after I had been stung on the arm by multiple paper wasps. The inflammation and pain persisted for months until my osteopath suggested I try bentonite clay as a poultice. It took several treatments to eliminate the toxins, but the pain and inflammation eventually disappeared!

Toxins come in a variety of forms and we may encounter some of them daily. They include paint, cleaning supplies, unpurified water, and pesticides (widely sprayed and left as residue on our fruits and vegetables). And then there are the toxins associated with a less-than-healthy diet and poor quality processed foods. Bentonite clay helps rid the body of these toxins, drawing them out, thus enhancing your immune system and reducing inflammation, as was the case with my paper wasp stings. The added benefit of bentonite clay is that it is not only a drawing agent but is also loaded with minerals essential to good health: calcium, magnesium, silica, sodium, copper,

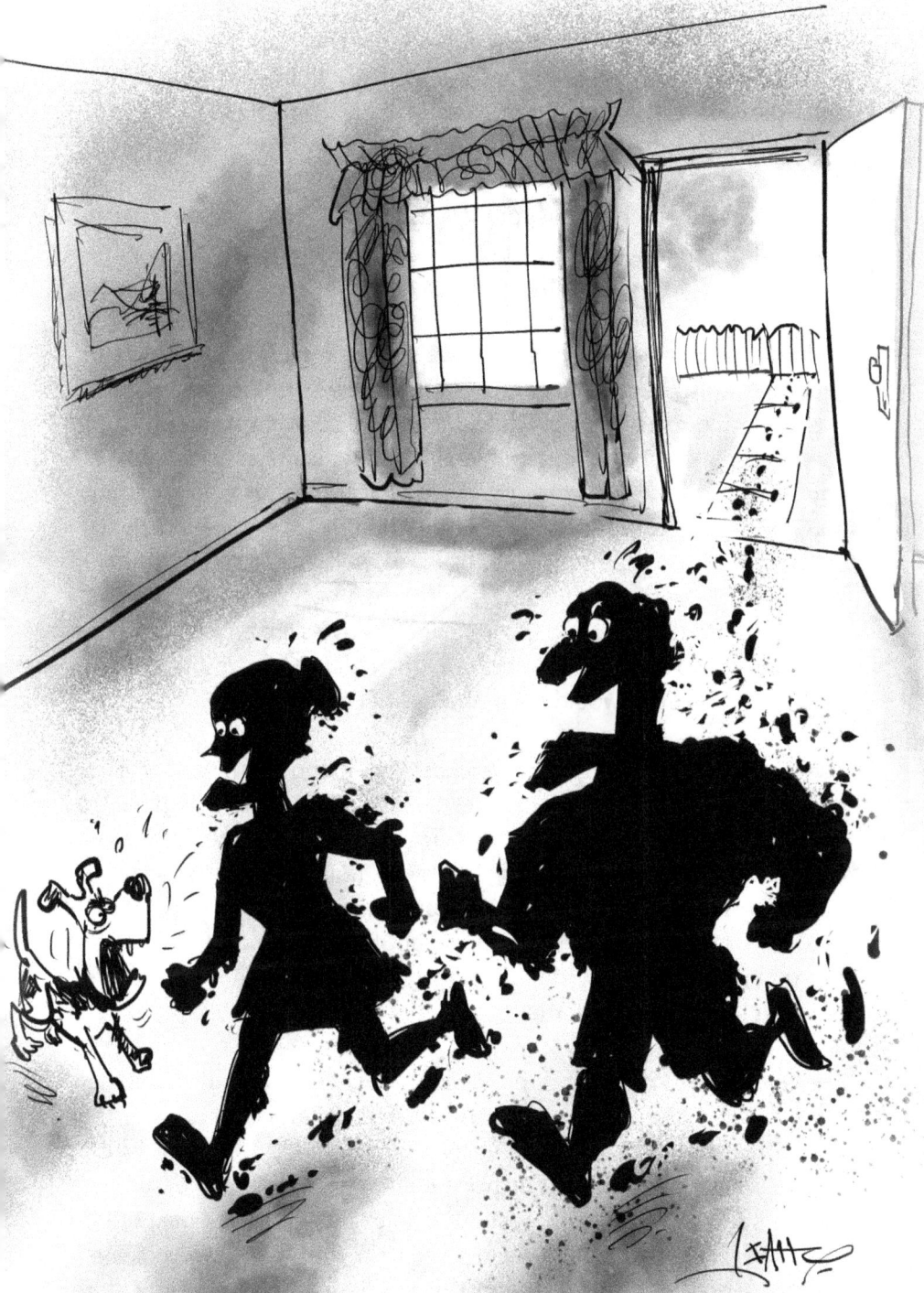

iron, and potassium to name a few. Bentonite clay has negatively charged molecules, while toxins are positively charged: the two bind and your body's elimination process takes it from there to rid your body of the nasties. The benefits are many.

For external use, create a poultice using one part clay, two parts water, and mix into a creamy paste. (Make sure you don't allow the clay to come in contact with metal, as this reduces its effectiveness.) Apply to your skin to aid in the healing of eczema, dermatitis, psoriasis, and other skin disorders. It's excellent for bites, cuts and stings (as I discovered). Just wrap the area covered in clay with wet gauze, cloth or plastic wrap. You can add it to your bath water or foot spa to dispel the toxins from your skin. Use it as a face mask – this is one of my favourite ways to use the clay. It leaves your skin smooth and hydrated and reduces any inflammation. It also oxygenates your cells, making you feel more energised, as well as supporting muscle recovery (Wellness Mama, 2017). But remember to remove the clay once it has dried, especially if you have sensitive skin, or you'll end up temporarily red-faced as I discovered when I left it on for longer than necessary, thinking I would maximise the benefits!

Used orally, the clay is an excellent oral rinse and teeth whitener to re-mineralise. Wellness Mama has an easy recipe for toothpowder if you'd like to try it (Wellness Mama, 2017a). For improved digestion and enhanced energy, take ½ teaspoon of the clay in a cup of water. Put it in a sealed container and shake well. You'll get most benefits from the clay without interference from other elements by taking it within an hour of food, or within two hours of medication and supplements.

The clay is also known to support pets that are unwell or vomiting. Mix in their water or dispense with an eye dropper.

You may have concerns about trace elements of naturally occurring lead in bentonite clay, and most companies list it on their packaging due to legislation. There is lead present in the clay, however, it is minimal. For instance, the brand I use is Redmond Clay from Utah in the United States, which has 11.9 parts per million (PPM) or 0.001190% per teaspoon. To put this in perspective and give you a comparison, according to the United States Environmental Protection Agency (EPA, 2017), the amount of lead in uncontaminated soil is between 50 to 400 PPM, which is considered safe. So, while containing trace elements of lead, bentonite clay is said to be safe to use in the dosages suggested, and the health benefits are enormous (Modern Alternative Health, 2017). Like Louis Litt, let's mud up!

58. Get a little dirty

Literally speaking. I was delighted when I came across this topic as a potential game-changer for better health, particularly with regard to children. It fitted so well with my innate understanding of the need for balance between a super-sterile world and one of squalor. In the developed world, we're bombarded with adverts pushing antibacterial this and that, cleaners that'll annihilate 99.99% of germs in our homes, supersonic disinfectants that immobilise the menacing microbes that lurk on every surface. Our obsession has come at a price, with an apparent seismic rise in inflammatory diseases such as asthma and allergies due, possibly, to a reduction in our exposure to microbes early in our lives. Allergies are a response to our immune systems getting out of control.

While on this topic, I acknowledge the ground-breaking work of German microbiologist, Robert Koch, who discovered in the late nineteenth century that bacteria was the cause of a range of infectious diseases, with the subsequent necessary sanitation and cleanliness that radically improved our health. It is essential that we wash our hands after bathroom visits and to maintain our personal hygiene regime. But have we become a little too clean for our own good? British epidemiologist, David Strachan, mooted an idea back in 1989 that he termed the 'hygiene hypothesis', the overzealousness for cleanliness, suggesting that exposure to infections as children would provide a defence against allergies later in life, helping build immunity against disease. Denis Kasper and his colleagues at Harvard Medical School undertook a study of germ-free and microbe-exposed mice in 2012 and discovered that the germ-free mice were susceptible to two immune diseases, asthma and ulcerative colitis. The results suggested that exposing mammals to bacteria relatively early in life built their resistance to these diseases (Chung *et al,* 2012). While the study cautions against making generalisations in applying these findings to humans, it fits the 'hygiene hypothesis' whereby an increase in inflammatory diseases in our developed world may be correlated to reduced exposure to microbes early in our lives.

Katia Moskvitch draws on the wisdom of epidemiologists, microbiologists and biologists to provide some ways we might navigate between the good and bad bacteria in our world. These suggestions include eating a varied diet preferably from farm produce; exercising outdoors rather than in a gym; digging in the garden; washing our hands stringently, but not washing our bodies excessively because this could disrupt the normal flora that keeps us healthy by competing with harmful organisms; timely cleaning rather than excessive cleaning around the house; closing the toilet lid when flushing to minimise the spread and multiplication of bacteria; allowing children to play among the soil and vegetation which are rich in beneficial microbes (Moskvitch, 2015). I recall the hours spent as a child making mud pies. It was lots of fun and perhaps gave me that early immunity to inflammatory diseases. While I couldn't find any evidence to connect an early life of microbe exposure to the centenarians I've drawn on for this book, I would imagine that many if not most grew up in a less sterile and less disinfected world. Could one of the secrets to their longevity be an exposure to a range of bacteria in early life that held them in good stead into their older years? Whatever the answer, these findings suggest a sensible balance of exposing ourselves to the good bacteria, while avoiding the bad bacteria, especially young children whose future health may very well depend upon it. To borrow and bend a comment erroneously attributed to Marie Antoinette: let them eat dirt! In light of the above, perhaps it's okay to let your kids lick the public swing and plant a kiss on the dog.

59. Breastfeeding = better health for nursing mothers

For my women readers of child-bearing age who may be umming and ahhing about whether to breastfeed and if it is beneficial to mother and baby, please read on. No doubt, you've already learned of the health benefits to the newborn: breast milk has a high population of bacteria and virus-fighting cells which develops stronger immune systems. With stronger immunity, breastfed babies are less likely to develop asthma and allergies, while also being less prone to respiratory and ear infections.

Now for the good news for breastfeeding mums themselves. A study published in the *Journal of the American Heart Association* (Park, 2017) suggests that breastfeeding may lower the mother's risk of heart attack and stroke, these benefits still being reaped even a decade after giving birth. The study was a broad and longitudinal one involving 290,000 Chinese women over a 10-year period. While the study points to an association between breastfeeding and lower heart disease risk, it does not infer that women who don't breastfeed will necessarily develop heart conditions. Nonetheless, the theory behind the findings is that breastfeeding reduces the metabolic reserves (body fat) that have accumulated during pregnancy, which in turn leads to lower risk factors of heart disease such as atherosclerosis and cholesterol.

60. Timely breast checks can save your life

Breast cancer is the most commonly diagnosed cancer in women in Australia, with eight women dying from the disease each day. It's estimated that the number of new cases in 2018 will be 18,087 women and 148 men! Yes, men are vulnerable too but statistically less likely to contract the disease. Of those numbers, 3,128 women and 28 men will die during the 2018 year. It's a bleak subject with dismal statistics, but extremely worthy of time and space here. The 'good news' in all this is that the survival rate for breast cancer is 90% and much of this is attributed to early detection (Cancer Australia, 2017). That's where you women and men come in. Early intervention with monthly self-examinations and periodic breast checks could mean the difference between life and death. And life is what this book is all about. The key to early breast cancer detection, according to Breast Cancer Network Australia (2018), is definitely self-examination because this regular process helps you to know your breasts well. We've all got a unique look and feel to our breasts: some lumpy, perhaps one is larger than the other, they come in a range of shapes and sizes, inverted nipples are a possibility either from birth or nursing, and so on. By looking and feeling, you'll recognise any changes from your norm. Check your breasts each month just after a shower, when applying body lotion or when you're getting dressed. For menstruating women, the ideal time is a week after your period. During menstruation, your breasts can naturally become lumpy so it's best to avoid the days prior to and following your menstrual cycle. You'll be checking all areas of your breasts with the flat pads of your three middle fingers, moving in small circular motions and checking the breasts, armpits and up to the collarbone.

What are you looking for with your self-examination? Symptoms and signs include new lumps in the breast or armpit area; thickening or swelling of your breast; any irritation or dimpling in the region; redness or flakiness of the skin around the nipple; puckering or pain around the nipple; discharge (other than breast milk for lactating mums); changes in the shape and size; or any persistent or unusual pain in the area of your breasts (Breast Cancer Network Australia, 2018). Most variations in the look and feel of your breasts are generally innocent, however, it's advisable to see your doctor if you discover any changes just to eliminate the possibility of something more sinister. As a follow-up to your own self-examination, free breast screenings are available through BreastScreen Australia for women aged 40 to 74, with 500 mobile units available across urban, rural and remote areas of Australia. For women younger than 40, the breast tissue is too dense to easily detect any cancers and statistically, women over 50 account for 75% of breast cancer cases. While a family history of breast cancer can play a part in increasing the risk of developing the disease, the percentage is relatively low with less than 5% associated with family history.

There are a few fundamental strategies you can adopt to minimise the risk of breast cancer. It's important to maintain a healthy body weight, have a daily activity/exercise regime, eat healthy foods including fruits and vegetables, avoiding processed foods, and limit your alcohol intake or cut alcohol out completely, especially if you have a family history of breast cancer (Cancer Council Australia, 2017). There's an excellent little three-minute British video clip that demonstrates how to undertake your self-examination. Cheekily called Coppafeel, it is part of a promotion run by a registered charity in the United Kingdom, and well worth the few minutes of your time (Coppafeel, 2018).

Many of us have probably known someone who has been diagnosed with breast cancer and perhaps some of those near and dear to us have, sadly, died as a result. Let's be super-vigilant with timely breast checks and a healthy lifestyle so we can live that long and healthy life we'd wish for ourselves and others.

61. Eradicate toxic chemicals from your bathroom

Did you know that many of our commercially available personal care products contain toxic chemicals that are making us sick? I have a pocket guide to toxins in the bathroom which I keep buried in my handbag. It provides a colour-coded warning for the range of toxic chemicals in our everyday personal care products: red (linked to cancer), orange (contaminated with carcinogens), green (skin or eye irritant), yellow (chemical toxins accumulating in organs), blue (known to cause respiratory problems), black (neurotoxins that damage the central nervous system — teratogen which affects the embryo, mutagen which induces genetic mutation).

Unlike Dorothy's experience in *The Wizard of Oz*, this rainbow of colours does not represent a land where all your dreams come true — more like nightmares! So, when I go shopping I'll check if any of the chemicals listed in the pocket guide are included in the product I'm considering purchasing. (Note: you may need a magnifying glass or a good pair of specs to read some of the elements listed in small font.)

Do you remember when your grandmother or great-grandmother used to use simple products such as baking soda and white vinegar for a range of personal care and cleaning alternatives? Well, I think it's time to return to those simpler days and rescue your health into the bargain. For instance, commercially available toothpaste contains fluoride, SLS saccharin, propylene glycol, artificial flavours and colours: most of these ingredients are dangerous. But do not despair, there are healthy and effective alternatives. For instance, baking soda makes an excellent toothpaste, and if you want to add a couple of drops of peppermint essential oil, you'll have white teeth and a fresh breath without any toxic risks. And it's probably a lot cheaper too! A large, smooth crystal of potassium aluminium sulphate makes a great alternative to commercially available antiperspirants. The toxic variety contains aluminium chlorohydrate, which is marked as red, yellow and blue on the pocket guide, whereas the crystal alternative contains larger molecule aluminium that is thought to be non-absorbent to the skin. Simply wet the crystal and apply as you would a regular roll-on deodorant. If you're wanting to eliminate aluminium completely, then you could search online for natural deodorants without that element.

I've included a link to Proactive Health in the *Reference List* with an image of a bathroom pocket guide that will help you identify the toxins in some commercially available personal care and household products. There are loads of safe and inexpensive remedies available online as well as links to non-toxic commercial products. My intention in this section is simply to bring your attention to potential health hazards of some commercially available products, so that you can enhance your health by choosing safer, cheaper alternatives (Proactive Health, nd).

62. Avoid chemically fragranced products

Unbelievably, many perfumes and colognes are not only intoxicating, they are also toxic. Most scented cosmetics contain petroleum-based chemicals known as phthalates. In the section in this book titled *Avoid heating foods in plastics* I explain that phthalates are a synthetic oil that wreaks havoc on the hormones. Due to trade-secret laws that protect perfume and cosmetic makers from divulging the specific formulas for their scents, there is no determining what specific chemicals are included. Phthalates keep the perfume's liquid elements suspended and distributed evenly, a chemical that Heid (2015) has also identified as disrupting our hormones. Famed Australian author, Kate Grenville, published *The Case Against Fragrance* in 2017, detailing her experience with fragrance sensitivity and how it has affected her health and wellbeing. What she includes as toxic fragrances goes well beyond perfumes: candles, air fresheners, deodorisers, and many perfumed cleaning products top the list of problem fragrances. According to a University of Melbourne study (Nourished Life, 2017), 33% of people are negatively impacted by fragrances and we're bombarded from all directions: air fresheners in offices, colleagues' perfumes and aftershaves, scented detergents and so on. Symptoms include headaches, migraines, nausea, and dry eyes. Asthma attacks are another side effect of exposure to fragrances.

Perhaps it's time to swap to natural and organic fragrances to smell sweet and live long. Just do an internet search on 'natural alternatives to toxic perfumes' and you'll find much on the web to intoxicate without the toxins. If you're considering disposing of those old perfumes from the back of the bathroom cabinet, they'll probably need to be decanted, the empty bottles sent to the recycling bin and the perfume liquid that you've collected taken to a toxic waste site. My perfume bottles are still sitting in my cupboard, but I have good intentions when the opportunity arises to get rid of them environmentally.

63. Pesticide detox to prevent Parkinson's disease

One of my all-time favourite singer/songwriters, Neil Diamond, was diagnosed with Parkinson's disease in 2018. Parkinson's is a degenerative disease of the central nervous system that primarily affects the motor system, so symptoms often include shaking, rigidity, slow movement, and difficulty walking. Diamond subsequently announced his retirement from touring (McMillen,

2018). His diagnosis is distressing news for the artist, his family and friends, and sad and crushing news for those of us who have listened to and loved Diamond's unique and wonderful music over many decades. His diagnosis spurred me to ask the question, just how pervasive is Parkinson's disease and are there natural, non-invasive ways to prevent it?

Others who have brought this disease into sharp relief in the past include professional boxer Muhammad Ali (now deceased), actor Michael J Fox and Olympic cyclist Davis Phinney, to name a few. My research revealed how pervasive and debilitating the disease is. Currently there is no cure, but there are certainly remedies to help prevent it, and others to alleviate symptoms. I learned that around four in every 1,000 Australians has Parkinson's disease, with this number increasing to one in 100 if you're aged over 60. Currently, there are approximately 80,000 Australians living with the disease (Department of Health & Human Services Victoria, 2017).

In the United States, over a million people suffer from it, with one in every 90 people unaware they have it. There are a range of factors associated with Parkinson's including genetics, head trauma and environmental factors such as pesticides (Dolhun, 2018). While head trauma and genetics are outside the scope of my discussion here, I'd like to consider environmental factors such as pesticides and how they might be impinging on our health, especially in relation to the risk of developing Parkinson's disease, and what we can do about it.

Pesticides are pervasive in society, from the foods we eat, the water we drink, the air we breathe, to our homes. Once these chemicals reach our cells, they make their way to our nervous system. For those with Parkinson's, it's the basal ganglia located in the midbrain that is compromised: it plays an important part in our ability to move. Should toxins infiltrate this region of the brain, dopamine is compromised, and cell death occurs (Sveinbjornsdottir, 2016). While avoiding chemicals and toxins altogether is not always practical or achievable, we can take measures to avoid an accumulation of them in our bodies with a few easy and non-invasive steps.

Eating fermented foods that keep the gut flora happy and healthy – which I've mentioned elsewhere for good health – is a great way to eradicate the pesticides. Kimchi, a favoured Korean dish, is loaded with good bacteria like lactobacilli. A 2010 study found that kimchi breaks down, degrades and totally eradicates the insecticide chlorpyrifos (Islam *et al,* 2010). Milk thistle is another wonderful chemical detox that can be taken in tea or supplement form. Cilantro (aka coriander on this side of the Pacific Ocean) is an aromatic annual of the parsley family and is excellent as a detoxifier of heavy metals, mercury and other toxic chemicals, working with your liver to remove these nasties. You can make a herbal tea or purchase it in liquid form. Wheatgrass offers another way to remove pesticides from the body and can be juiced along with all your other lovely vegetables (see the heading *Vegetable juicing* in this book). But start with small amounts of wheatgrass, as it is a powerful detoxing agent!

There are also simple things like regular exercise to increase blood circulation, and jumping in a sauna or jacuzzi to sweat out those grubby pesticides and toxins. Remember not to overdo the heat and steam and to stay hydrated.

Finally, there's my old faithful go-to – fibre, especially in the form of organic vegetables and fruits. Fibre is like a street sweeper for your digestive system, picking up all the rubbish along the way and sending it packing (Natural On, 2018).

There are several other ways to eliminate pesticides, which you can find at the Natural On website (follow the link in the *Reference List* at the end of this book). If you make just one of these strategies part of your health regime, then you are certainly supporting yourself towards better health and perhaps reducing your chances of becoming one of the 80,000 people in Australia currently with Parkinson's.

64. Butt out

I'm not telling you to mind your own business, I'm referring to cigarette smoking and passive (second-hand) smoking. If you're a smoker, you must clearly care about your health and want to do something to improve it. God love you and good on you! The biggest favour you can do for your body and your health is to put that butt out for the final time and never touch the smokes again. Did you know that in an Australian study, it was revealed that smoking was the leading preventable cause of disease in 2003 and that 15,500 people lost their lives in that year as a direct result of smoking (Australian Government Department of Health, 2018)?

As a former smoker, I know how difficult it can be to quit, but quit you must if you want any chance of making your healthy 100 in this life. And it's not just your life that's at risk: others are passively inhaling your toxic fumes and they run the same risk of disease and mortality. Both smokers and passive smokers inhale the smoke and the toxins travel anywhere within the body where blood flows, causing harm to nearly every organ and system. Forget low-tar and low-nicotine cigarettes; they're just as poisonous. While you may not experience the adverse consequences of tobacco smoking immediately, you can 'look forward' to any or all of the following: a range of cancers, heart disease, stroke, atherosclerosis, abdominal aortic aneurysm, emphysema and other respiratory diseases, blindness, dental problems, erectile dysfunction, reduced fertility in women, osteoporosis, and pregnancy complications. Tobacco smoking is linked to more cancer deaths in Australia than any other factor (Powell, 2018). Tobacco contains 7,000 chemicals, more than 70 of which are carcinogenic. These cancer-causing agents include carbon monoxide (car exhaust fumes), ammonia (floor cleaner) and arsenic (rat poison). If I'm frightening you, good! It's important that you're rattled so that you absolutely know how you're compromising your health and the health and wellbeing of others around you.

According to a French study, smoking around children is responsible for the greater risk of their developing rheumatoid arthritis! And have I mentioned how detrimental it is to your looks? The aging process is said to accelerate in those who smoke cigarettes, so if you care about your appearance (as I do), then quitting is a no-brainer. There's lots of support out there to help you quit: willpower and going 'cold turkey' may not be enough. If you've tried going it alone and failed, then you could contact the Australian Government agency, QuitNow, through their website, or the helpline Quitline (Telephone 13 78 48). There's your local GP who'll be a wonderful source of wisdom on how to stop. There's also prescription medications available to help with the cravings and the effects of withdrawal. You can see your pharmacist about nicotine replacement therapy. Then there's hypnosis therapy to assist you to quit the habit, or other behavioural therapies. Whatever you decide, have a plan and stick to it. Perhaps have someone keep you accountable until you're through the worst of it. E-cigarettes, or the practice known as 'vaping', may be a possible alternative to cigarette smoking for some. Ironically, vaping products are readily available in Australia, however, the nicotine liquid itself remains illegal here (Powell, 2018). While apparently less injurious to your health, e-cigarettes also have their risks with data suggesting vaping may pose harm to your immune system – and behavioural and reproductive risks to children of women who vape during pregnancy (Raloff, Science News, 2016). Also, evidence from a small study from Johns Hopkins released in 2018 suggests that the heating coils within e-cigarettes generate unsafe levels of lead, chromium, manganese, and/or nickel. Chronic inhaling of these metals is linked to respiratory and cardiovascular diseases as well as cancer (Johns Hopkins Bloomberg School of Public Health, 2018). So butt out – and vape out – to beat the beggar before it beats you and those around you (QuitNow, 2017; How to Quit Smoking, 2017).

65. Get some indoor plants

Having indoor plants was a trend in the 70s and 80s for decorating the home. The trend is now back, with benefits way beyond aesthetics. When you read what follows, you may well be as amazed as I was at how life-enhancing the humble indoor plant can be. It's been scientifically established that indoor plants help us live longer and healthier. For starters, our house plants can markedly improve our concentration and productivity, reduce our stress levels, elevate our mood, improve our respiratory health, and reduce our risk of cancer-related diseases (Lee, 2017). Scientists have long known that plants are adept at absorbing, through their leaves, gases such as carbon dioxide, an ability that enables photosynthesis. But it's the air-purification process where a house plant really comes into its own, absorbing harmful volatile organic compounds (VOCs) such as benzene sourced from plastics, fabrics, pesticides, and cigarette smoke, and formaldehyde derived from cosmetics, detergents, fabric softeners, and carpet cleaners. These nasty VOCs have been associated with asthma, nausea, respiratory complaints, and cancer (Palermo, 2013). House plants are miniature versions of forests, which are known as the 'lungs of the earth' for their ability to absorb carbon dioxide and produce oxygen, working to protect our planet's biodiversity. Researchers from Harvard's T H Chan School of Public Health conducted an eight-year study (2000–2008) using data from over 100,000 women on the association between vegetation and mortality rates. What they discovered was that the women who were surrounded by vegetation and plants had a 12% lower mortality rate than those living with less greenery around them. The study suggested that this link might also have contributed to the lower levels of depression (30%) among the 'green' women. Added to this was the women's lower rates for respiratory diseases (34%) and cancer (13%) compared with those with no vegetation around their homes (Datz, 2016).

Some of the best plants for your home include orchids, succulents, snake plants, and bromeliads, especially ideal in the bedroom as most other plants emit oxygen during the day and carbon dioxide at night when the photosynthesis process has stopped. These little gems do the opposite, emitting oxygen at night – excellent for better sleep. If you're new to plants around the house, succulents are a great start as they're low maintenance, hardy and suited to most homes. They like some sunlight, so a windowsill is a good place for them (Lee, 2017). Chatting to the wise plant folk at your local nursery might be a good way to start greening your way to good health. If you want to live longer, then perhaps it's time to turn over a new leaf.

66. Gardening and pottering can save your life

According to a university hospital in Stockholm, heart attacks and strokes were reduced by 27% in a 12-year study of 4,232 individuals. These folks ditched their sedentary lifestyle for a more active one and among the activities was gardening and pottering around the house. Of course, it's important that it be something you enjoy doing. As long as the activity involves getting your body a little warmer, breathing a little harder and having an elevated heart rate – which gardening and other DIY activities invoke – then you're on your way to a healthier lifestyle. While this study focused on the over-60s, there's no reason to believe that this approach wouldn't also be beneficial for anyone throughout their lives, as a way of reducing cardiovascular disease.

Now, where's that shovel and those gardening gloves?

67. Avoid heating foods in plastics

I tried to come up with a humorous spin on this topic, but I figured because of its serious nature, it was best to put out the warning rather than make light of it. As mentioned elsewhere in this book, the Canadian environmental scientists Bruce Lourie and Rick Smith (ABC Radio, 2013), conducted an experiment in which they deliberately poisoned themselves with exposure to plastic chemicals, all in the name of science. They discovered that with our exposure to plastics in our everyday lives (especially when coming in contact with heat), toxic chemicals are released into our bodies. Among the chemicals is one known as phthalates. Phthalates are a synthetic oil that wreaks havoc on the hormone system.

Lourie and Smith provide suggestions for avoiding this harmful chemical, including not heating your food in plastic in the microwave, avoiding non-stick frypans for cooking and checking the recycling number on plastic toys. The safe numbers are 4, 5, 1, and 2. The numbers to avoid are 7 and 3 – both contain harmful chemicals. Buying foods in glass containers rather than plastic containers is another way to avoid exposure. They suggest that the epidemic proportions of autism, ADHD, asthma, and obesity have very strong correlations to exposure to these harmful phthalates. While I still have plastics in my cupboard, I don't use them for heating of any kind. I still use them for leftovers and for freezing foods. I now have a non-Teflon pan for cooking. Glass and ceramic ware are my new best friends in the kitchen, as are wooden or metal stirring spoons for cooking. Lourie and Smith also warn of the risks of using antibacterial chemicals or products that are highly fragrant, which would suggest the presence of phthalates. The scientists argue that it's not the one-off use of these products, but a lifetime of exposure that causes the problems, and exposure to the developing brains of young children.

68. Digital detoxing and electromagnetic radiation reduction

Quite a mouthful, isn't it! But it's a serious issue worthy of consideration. Firstly, let's consider the 'data deluge' that surrounds and pervades our lives. The digital world as we know it started back in the 1970s with the introduction of personal computers. Smartphones emerged in the mid-1990s with Apple iPhones launching in 2007, followed by Android smartphones in 2009. As of 2018, there were 2.53 billion smartphones globally, predicted to grow to around 2.9 billion by 2019 (Statista, 2018)! With such a pervasive uptake and cultural embrace of this technology, it's important to understand the health implications.

If you're serious about good health, then you need to take some time away from the smartphone, the iPad, the laptop, or the desktop computer. There are loads of great strategies available to help you break your addiction to constant Facebook or Instagram checks. Neen James (2017) offers 10 top tips for 'detoxing' from your digital devices. James suggests you start with a specific time frame: if you're totally addicted to your devices, start with, say, three hours. Next, let your family and friends know of your detoxing and that you won't be available electronically for a period of time. You'll need to put your devices away somewhere, so you won't be tempted to check. Turn your devices off or turn the sound off so the message notifications won't lure you back. Apple Inc. have also recognised the need for digital detoxing with the release of a new screen time initiative for digital health, software that helps monitor and limit the time spent on your iPhones and tablets (The Verge, 2018). James (2017) further suggests doing something that you've been putting off: it can be pleasurable, say, reading a real book that you've been given as a gift but haven't yet read. If you're engaged with the technology but don't want additional distractions, there's blocking software such as Freedom App that will block websites so you can get things done. Another strategy is simply going for a quiet walk outdoors to be alone with your thoughts. The author also advocates scheduling some fun while detoxing. What would you love to do that doesn't involve technology? Let someone know that you'll be offline to help keep you accountable in your digital detox phase. Finally, focus on a project, or a conversation, or spend time with your family and friends. Eye-to-eye contact is a wonderful antidote to digital toxins.

Having discussed the *addictive* effects of our digital technologies and how to address them, it's also important to consider the possible *toxic* effects of the digital world. With the advent of wireless devices, there has been an exponential increase in radiofrequency (RF) exposure, along with hypersensitivity and diseases associated with electromagnetic field (EMF) and RF exposure. Additionally, exposure is amplified by cellular data network connections, Wi-Fi connectivity, Bluetooth emitters, and GPS tracking. While studies have produced conflicting results on RF radiation and illness, prolonged exposure to smartphone radiation cannot be beneficial to our health and wellbeing. In fact, what follows would suggest there is a school of thought on their risks to our health. Cell Wellbeing (2017) comprises an international and multidisciplinary team of highly qualified experts in epigenetics, naturopathy and nutrition. This team argues that there are negative consequences to the exposure we're experiencing in our digital world. Professor Emeritus Martin Pall (2013), a member of the Cell Wellbeing team, argues that the advent of wireless devices in particular has caused a huge increase in RF exposure resulting in hypersensitivity and diseases related to EMF and RF exposure. Pall (2017) claims that diseases associated with prolonged exposure to EMFs and RFs include cancer, neurological disease, reproductive disorders, immune dysfunction, and electromagnetic hypersensitivity.

But there are some simple solutions to offset the health challenges in our wired and wireless world. For instance, sleeping with the mobile phone away from the bedside table, and using loudspeaker and hands-free options rather than holding the phone to your ear. Switching off the Wi-Fi modem at night and using waveform harmonisers that clean up the air pollutants is another effective strategy. Drinking good quality water, eating healthily, taking walks in the countryside to ground yourself, and supplementing with minerals and antioxidants will collectively help you to detoxify your body of RFs and EMFs.

From a nutritional perspective, health coach Dr Thomas Bige (personal communication, 6 October 2016) recommends high calcium foods to protect from calcium depletion caused by EMF exposure. These foods include salmon, sardines, dark green leafy vegetables, almonds, asparagus, blackstrap molasses, brewer's yeast, broccoli, cabbage, carob, kale, mustard greens, figs, soybeans, tofu, watercress, chickweed, chicory, flaxseed, kelp, parsley, sesame seeds, and poppy seeds. Along with drinking good quality water, Bige recommends incorporating essential fatty acids into the diet. These are derived from salmon, mackerel, sardines, herring, trout, flaxseed, walnuts, pumpkin seeds, hemp seeds, and soybeans. These essential fatty-acid sources strengthen the cell membrane against the effects of EMFs.

69. Use a squatty potty

A *what*, you ask? A squatty potty is a device you can position in front of a standard toilet, elevating your legs and resulting in a squat rather than a sitting position when defecating. It also tucks away easily at the base of your toilet when not in use. Why is squatting better than sitting? you might be pondering. The answer is simple. When we sit to poop, the puborectalis muscle (rectum) creates a natural kink that ensures faecal continence. Squatting relaxes this muscle for easier elimination of your poop. It is also theorised that easier elimination results in a cleaner colon which leads to a healthier colon.

German scientist Guilia Enders (2016) has a special interest in the human gastrointestinal tract and the importance of squatting for good bowel health. Enders says that squatting to poop results in fewer incidences of diverticulosis and haemorrhoids. Furthermore, Enders states that the seated style for defecation favoured by much of the Western world can raise the risk of varicose veins, stroke and defecation syncope (fainting while on the toilet). So, when you've got to go, place your feet on your squatty potty, incline your body slightly forward and pass your motion with ease. While conceding that the stool (pardon the pun) doesn't allow for a full squat, this partial squatting position does open up the colon for easier evacuation. Now, that's a relief! (Ho, 2016; Squatty Potty, 2018).

70. Poop patrol

While discussing poop, it is opportune to chat about the importance of *checking* your poo. I'll also offer some other insights around faecal matter. This may not be a subject you find appealing, but awareness around any atypical stools could alert you to early signs of infection or other serious conditions, prompting you to consult your medical professional. Several years ago, I came across the Bristol Stool Chart, a medical aid designed to classify faeces into seven groups (Heaton & Lewis, 1997: 920-924). The time that faeces remain in the colon often determines the type of stool. By the time it gets to the toilet bowl, it will reveal a lot about you and your health. Your stools are influenced by the foods you eat, the fluids you drink, any medications and supplements you take, and your lifestyle. You can use the Bristol Stool Chart to check what your stools are telling you. Type 1, for example, is described as separate hard lumps; type 2 indicate sausage-shaped, lumpy faeces. These first two types, unsurprisingly, indicate constipation. Type 3 is sausage-like with cracks. Type 4 is also sausage- or snake-like, smooth and soft. Types 3 and 4 are referred to as the perfect poo, as they're soft and easier to pass. Types 5 to 7 range from soft blobs, mushy to watery or entirely liquid. These, again unsurprisingly, suggest diarrhoea and – more seriously – perhaps a need to seek medical attention, especially for Type 7 (Continence Foundation of Australia, 2018). But texture and shape are not the only considerations when analysing your poop: the colour of the stool is also a consideration. Your normal poop may be many shades of brown, although ingesting supplements, medications and dark foods and fruits might manifest as black or dark green stools. While poop is generally an unpleasant odour, particularly strong or foul-smelling stools could indicate that all is not well in the state of your colon (Humana, 2014). In any case, it is wise to consult your medical professional about any concerns you may have in this regard.

On a quirky but financially rewarding note, did you know that there's a thriving industry in selling your healthy poop? Faecal transplants are becoming an effective treatment for those with bacterial infections and other gut disorders, often associated with prolonged use of antibiotics. They're also becoming more common in treating conditions such as irritable bowel syndrome, chronic fatigue, Parkinson's, and autism (Asher, 2017). This is not a new phenomenon: faecal transplants have been around in the west since the 1950s, and the Chinese have been practising the art since the fourth century. However, it is only relatively recently that Western studies have revealed the therapeutic potential around stools (Aroniadis & Brandt, 2013). If you are deemed an ideal donor, your healthy poop is collected, put through a blender and inserted into the bowel of a patient with poor or diminished gut bacteria. The theory is that the healthy microbiota in your stools will inhabit the colon of the recipient, and *voila*, a healthier gut.

In Australia, the Melbourne Faecal Microbial Transplant organisation offers donors and recipients information about this procedure. Donating your healthy faecal matter may not lead to a longer life for *you*, but it's another good reason to follow a healthy lifestyle because your donations could well support others to greater health. There's the wonderful story of 18-year-old Australian girl, Rachel Challen, who suffered from a severe bowel condition and her father's healthy poop came to the rescue. A faecal microbiota transplant ultimately saved her life (Stevenson, 2016).

There is, however, a cautionary note with regard to faecal transfers, especially for the recipients. It is well known that the state of your gut impacts either positively or negatively on your mood, sleep and stress levels. This is because there is a bidirectional (two-way) relationship with your central nervous system, referred to as the 'gut-brain axis', whereby the gut sends and receives messages from the brain (The Conversation, 2018). Research has found that faecal transplants can cause the recipients of the transfers to adopt the physical and mental traits of the donors. Associate Professor Patrick Charles from the Department of Infectious Diseases at Austin Health stated that "the change in the mix of bacteria when you get this transplant can alter the person who is getting it to take on some of the characteristics of the donor sometimes... There have been people who have taken on the shape of the donor, such as if the donor is either overweight or underweight they've become more like that". And Charles goes on to argue that people who've never experienced depression may experience depression after the transplant (Asher, 2013). Reassuringly for recipients, there are stringent health criteria to be met by donors before samples can be used.

If you intend donating, it is wise to notify the faecal bank of any physical or emotional conditions you have. The science around the transfer of physical and emotional traits from donor to recipient is relatively uncharted waters. I wonder if the inverse could be true; could donors who are physically and emotionally well in certain areas help recipients who are unwell in these areas? Exciting and interesting times ahead for poop.

71. Take a daily 15–20 minute nap

You're probably muttering to yourself that taking a daily nap is not always practical or possible, especially if you work full time or have other daytime commitments. However, the benefits of a little daily snooze are remarkable and can, in some circumstances, save your life, as you'll discover. Some of the greatest-ever minds such as Albert Einstein and Thomas Edison included a daily nap in their lives. Other famous nappers include Leonardo Da Vinci, Margaret Thatcher, Bill Clinton, Eleanor Roosevelt, and actress Emmy Rossum, to name but a few (Hall, 2014). These notable nappers are fine examples of the scientific understanding that 40 winks can reverse the brain-aging process. According to Dr Manolis Kallistratos of the European Society of Cardiology, taking a midday nap is associated with lower blood pressure and a reduction in the need for some hypertension medications. The former means that there's less pressure on the arteries and heart, while the latter is associated with the probability of fewer drugs due to a lower BP (2015).

But we need look no further than centenarian Flossie Dickey of Washington State who lived to be 110 years and 279 days. On her hundred and tenth birthday, she told reporters that she napped often and also enjoyed a whiskey straight up (Shah, 2016). A shot of whiskey may or may not be an appropriate accompaniment to your daily snooze (especially if you're at work) but I'd like to think that Flossie's napping habit was one reason for her longevity.

There are various approaches to napping, as outlined by sleep specialist Damiana Corca (2016).

Firstly, there's your typical 15–20-minute daily nap which is most effective when taken routinely and at a regular time each day. This type of napping is also an excellent antidote for the insomniac, as exhaustion (following a sleepless night) can often inhibit the ability to fall asleep.

A power nap is another important form of napping. If you have a big function in the evening or even a daytime activity that'll require your full attention, a planned snooze without necessarily feeling tired might just be the tonic for you.

Then there's the more obvious life-saving kind of nap. Driving while fatigued is a killer, and you need emergency napping time. Pulling over to the side of the road in a safe place and having a recovery rest will literally save your life and re-energise you for the travel ahead.

Our feline companions are masters in the art of catnapping. Perhaps it's one of the reasons cats are said to have nine lives. We may not be able to compete with the snoozing ability of our furry friends, but we can do this one little thing to live a longer, healthier life. Give yourself permission to take a little snooze each day. Fifteen minutes makes you more productive and energised and adds life to your years, and years to your life. The catchcry here is: you snooze, you win!

72. Undertake a first aid course in CPR training (a life saver)

While this tip won't necessarily save *your* life, it could save the life of a stranger or someone near and dear to you who may have experienced some kind of trauma leading to cardiac arrest. For instance, cessation of breathing or heartbeat can occur after an electric shock, a drowning or heart attack among many other factors. The shocking statistics are that 30,000 Australians suffer from a cardiac arrest each year and only 10% of those people survive! In Seattle, cardiopulmonary resuscitation (CPR) training is mandated in primary schools and also before acquiring a driver's licence. The survival rate for a witnessed cardiac arrest in Seattle is 62%.

If the heart suddenly stops beating and nothing is done, you're brain-damaged in four minutes and after 10 minutes, you're unlikely to survive. With an average response time for an ambulance in Australia being nine minutes, those in the immediate vicinity of a casualty are more likely to be the ones who can save the casualty's life if they know CPR. When I renewed my CPR recently, the St John's Ambulance instructor reminded our group of those vital four minutes after a person stops breathing. Brain damage or death can occur after that precious four minutes has elapsed because there's no flow of blood to the vital organs and so the body begins to shut down. Time is critical. Unless the incident occurs within a medical setting, no ambulance or medical team is likely to be on hand and if you are willing and able, then you have the opportunity to render first aid and perhaps revive an otherwise dying casualty. In some parts of the world a bystander has a responsibility to render first aid.

The St John program follows the DRSABCD process.

D is for danger to self and the casualty and others. It's so important that you don't become a casualty yourself in your bid to help someone else, so use all your senses to determine that it is safe for you to approach an unconscious casualty.

R is for response. Here, you'll be checking for any reactions from the casualty so look, listen and feel.

S reminds you to send for help. In Australia, you or someone else near you can call triple zero (000) or 112 to advise where you are, the facts about the casualty's state and the circumstances.

A is for airway. Check the casualty's airway for any obstructions by turning them on their side and scooping out any obstructions. (Ideally, you would wear gloves for protection.) Once cleared, return the casualty onto their back then tilt their head back to open the airway.

B is for breathing. If they're not breathing, then you begin **C**, which refers to CPR. Your course instructor will train you in how to locate the exact position for undertaking CPR, depending on whether it is a baby, a child or an adult, and the depth of the compressions which is roughly one-third the depth of the chest. CPR has been simplified over the years and the agreed process is now 30 chest compressions followed by two rescue breaths. You'll need to continue this process for two minutes (or about four rotations of 30 x 2) before checking for breathing. If no breathing, repeat the chest compressions and breaths until help arrives or the casualty commences breathing.

D is for defibrillator. For an unconscious adult who is not breathing, apply an automated external defibrillator (AED) if available. AEDs are routinely found in many public places including large shopping centres, clubs and other organisations. They're designed to deliver an electric shock for irregular heart rhythm (arrhythmia) in order to re-establish a normal heartbeat. AEDs are simple to operate. Just follow the automated voice prompts. If the casualty responds to defibrillation, then turn them onto their side with head tilted to maintain an airway and await medical help.

I cannot stress how effective it is to physically go through the processes of CPR. You will feel much more confident about making the decision to offer life-saving resuscitation. There are numerous stories circulating on the internet of people being revived with this immediate first aid response. You can also download the St John Ambulance Australia First Aid app to your iPhone for easy access to the knowledge in case you're a little unsure. I'm sharing this 'health' tip with you because I firmly believe that the more people who are trained in first aid, the safer, more resilient and longer living our communities will be.

73. Pet ownership

Owning a pet leads to a healthier you. There are an estimated 25 million pets in the homes, back yards and farms of Australians (Ringland, 2017). That's one pet for each of us, so perhaps I'm preaching to the converted with this topic. Nevertheless, I'll carry on just in case there's one or two of you who haven't caught the pet bug yet. Others may not know of the amazing health benefits. I appreciate that some of my readers may not be in a position to own a pet, but pets do come in many species and sizes to suit a variety of households and lifestyles. They range from reptiles such as lizards and snakes, to birds in cages, fluffy cats and kittens, and of course, the big buddy of this world, the dog!

According to RSPCA Australia, owning a pet has both physical and psychological benefits. A pet's presence in your life can improve

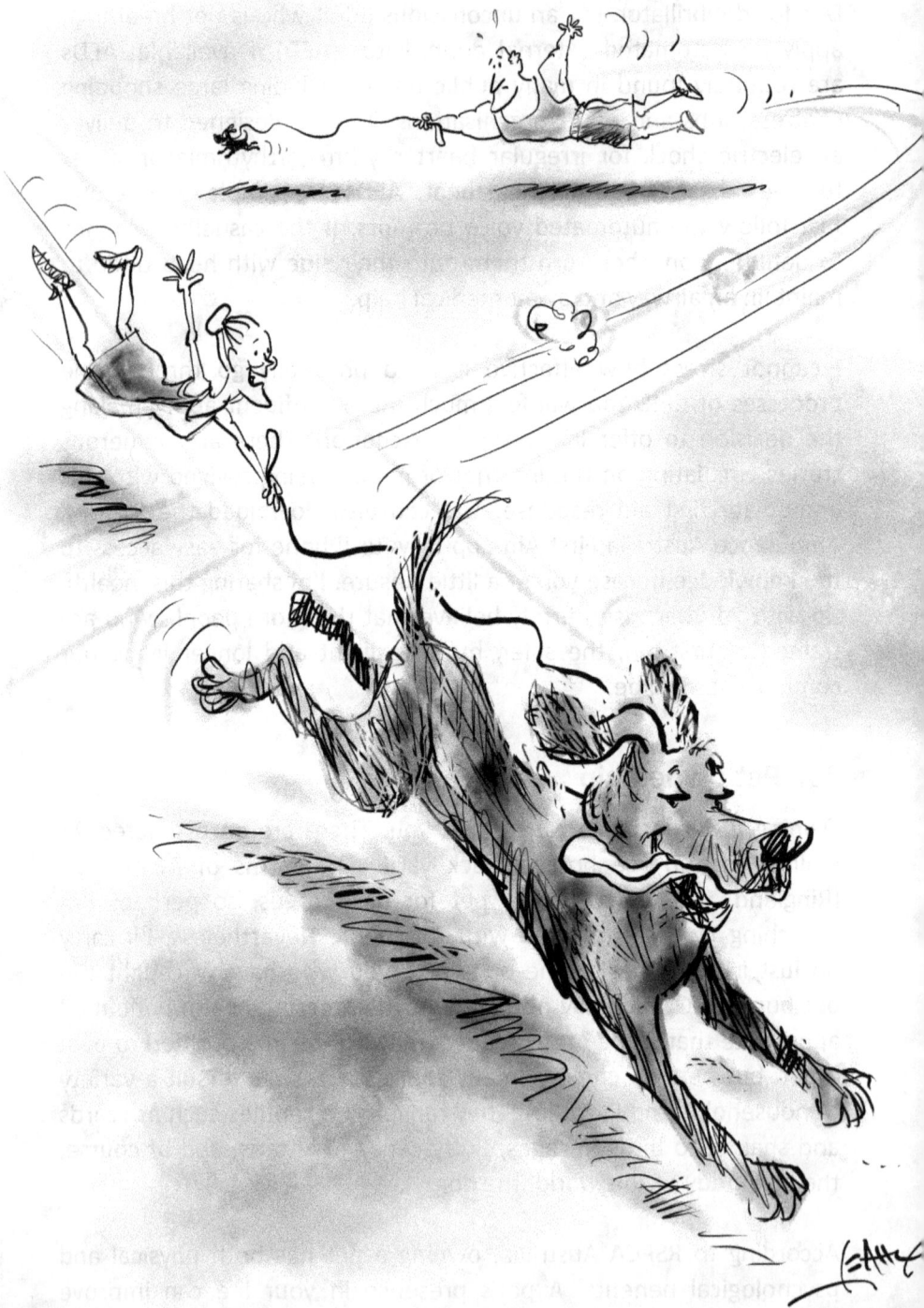

your cardiovascular wellbeing by lowering your blood pressure and cholesterol levels. Furthermore, you're more likely to engage in physical activity (especially with dog ownership) and this translates to fewer doctor visits. Aussies have one of the highest rates of pet ownership in the world. Dog and cat ownership has been associated with such positive influences that there is a yearly saving of $3.86 billion in health expenditure. The psycho-emotional benefits are just as marvellous: pet owners are said to be more empathetic and to have greater self-esteem; they're less likely to suffer depression and have greater coping abilities; and pet ownership creates opportunities for social connection. While owning a pet has its responsibilities, the rewards to your health and wellbeing seem more than worth it. If you're considering acquiring a pet, I recommend you look online at the RSPCA's Adopt-A-Pet website. They have so many adorable pets just waiting for their forever home. In helping yourself to reach a healthy 100, you're also helping save the life of a pet worth loving (RSPCA Australia, 2015).

If owning a pet is out of the question for one reason or another, there are always cat videos! It's a relatively recent craze that's been proven to boost mood and energy levels (Indiana University, 2015). As at 2017, by searching 'cat videos' you get about 161 million hits, with Grumpy Cat and Lil Bub among the most popular because of their unique appearance (Hill, 2017). With so much to choose from, there's bound to be one or two that'll do the trick. I dare you to watch a cat video and not feel good and be enthralled and energised. Where possible, the real thing is probably the best health tonic. The RSPCA here in Australia has a veritable Noah's Ark of animals to suit your lifestyle.

74. A daily five-minute dose of journalling

I read author and filmmaker Julia Cameron's book, *The Artist's Way* (2002), some years ago. Creativity is a way of life for her. Two basic tenets underpin her book. The first is the unlocking of our creativity through daily stream-of-consciousness journal writing. The second principle Cameron advocates is a creative expedition which she refers to as an 'artist's date' (a date with oneself) once a week to experience something that enchants or interests you, as a way of unlocking your creativity. I undertook the occasional artist's date, but more importantly I wrote those pages religiously each day for many years and experienced a level of creative inspiration. However, as the years progressed and my life became busier, I found the one-hour journalling commitment each morning onerous and time-consuming, so I dropped that long process. However, Cameron's basic tenet stayed with me: I recognised that daily journalling is a very good self-care process but that it needn't require more than five minutes of my day to still have powerful, positive effects.

Kriss Britton, from *I Heart Wellness* (2016) uses her daily five-minute journal as a way of dumping all the 'stuff' of life – confusion, anxiety, etc., as well as using her writing as a way of gaining clarity around issues. It has become a way of clearing her mind for greater peace, wellbeing and productivity. Britton makes the process appealing too. She suggests getting a fun journal that is visually appealing to make you want to write in it. She also recommends using a favourite pen. This daily dose of journalling has transformed her life and those of her many followers. Where once she had low self-worth, her writing helps her see the importance of self-care which she describes "like... breathing fresher air and your soul is alive". My own journalling clears my mind of all the chatter and frees me up to focus on the things that really matter in life. The sense of peace and wellbeing that your journalling can create offers you a simple tool for a daily dose of wellbeing and inspiration.

75. Under-whelm the overwhelm

The term 'overwhelm' has been around since the 1300s so it's not unique to our twentieth/twenty-first century lifestyle. With all the new and digital technologies we have around us, you'd think our workload would lessen, not increase. But that's exactly what has happened, leading many of us to feel a sense of overwhelm. The sources of overwhelm go beyond technologies. 'I'm feeling stressed and overwhelmed' is a disturbing catchcry because when you feel as if you've got the weight of the world on your shoulders, stress follows, and ill-health can often be just behind it. You may also feel a sense of stagnation and be unable to take any action at all. But do not despair because there are several proven strategies that work wonders in addressing those times when you're buried beneath a mass of small, large or terrifying things to do or address. A brilliant technique that's worked for me and others I've supported is to do a 'data dump': putting everything that is overwhelming you out of your head and onto the page. A large A3 sheet works best with a pen or pencil. There's no priority: just get it all out on paper, exhausting every big and little action or 'to do' that you have. Don't edit this phase – there's no right or wrong. If it's overwhelming you, it's important and it goes onto the page. If you need more than one A3 sheet, go for it. This is a terrific cleansing and calming process and you'll probably feel as though someone has lifted a load from your shoulders. They have, and that someone is you. Dr John Demartini ascribes to a similar process which he calls the 'Distraction Resolution Process' (2018). He recommends making lists of everything that occupies your mind or distracts you. However, Demartini adds some components to the process to reduce anxiety and uncertainty while increasing the probability of taking fulfilling action. Once your data dump or list has been accomplished, Demartini suggests you identify those items that can be done by others and then delegate accordingly, freeing you up to work on the actions within your particular expertise. Next, date all the items. You'll be surprised to find that not everything needs to be done today. You can then put them in your calendar for later action. This process will reveal your priority list.

Dr Libby Weaver (2016b: 283-285) offers a refinement of this calendar process. Weaver advocates scheduling actions/meetings/ to-dos into 15-minute intervals in your calendar. Her mantra is that 'if it doesn't get scheduled, it doesn't get done'. Once you have them in order, you may need to chunk them into manageable steps. You can then take each one individually and list seven high-priority action steps to fulfil each objective. At the close of each day, take a moment to check off those things you've achieved. The consequent reduction in anxiety, stress and tension will improve your digestive health too. The feeling of being more productive will lead to a greater sense of self-worth and accomplishment, and no doubt add years to your life and life to your years (Demartini, nd).

76. Don't sweat the small stuff

I read this sage advice while sitting in the waiting area at my chiropractor's. It was the title of a book sitting on the shelf among other health-related publications. The author, Richard Carlson, had a subtitle: ...and it's all small stuff (1997). I've been known to sweat the small stuff from time to time, and it was as if the book was speaking directly to me. I was intrigued. I began to leaf through some of Carlson's wisdom. Fortunately, my chiropractor was running behind time, so I managed to read quite a few pages before the receptionist called me. (The book was clearly working already, as I'm impatient yet I was oblivious to the time.) Later, I went online and ordered my own copy and couldn't put it down.

Carlson provides a myriad of ways to put things in perspective and prevent the little things in life from driving us crazy. Beyond that, he helped me reach beyond myself and redesign how to engage with others. He recalls seeing a bumper sticker, 'Practice Random Acts of Kindness and Senseless Acts of Beauty'. It was a profound piece of wisdom for me. I immediately organised a bumper sticker for my car with those very words. I don't know what other commuters think, but it is a great reminder to me, whenever getting into or out of my car, to put things in perspective each day, not worry about 'stuff' because it's all small and inconsequential in the big scheme of things, see 'stuff' as opportunities, and, at the end of each day, leave the world a better place.

Dr Libby Weaver (2013) also discusses this issue in her book *Beauty from the Inside Out,* from the perspective of how our perceptions can play a role in developing stress. Weaver provides some wonderful insights into how you might respond to the "undulations of life" and once more begin to "laugh at the calamity, the chaos, and the small stuff". Resting, diaphragmatic breathing and laughter are all wonderful strategies to put things back in perspective, Weaver argues, some of which I've discussed in more detail elsewhere in this book. My health coach, Dr Thomas Bige, made a sobering comment related to this topic when he commented on my tendency to hang onto things from my past: "You can't change the past, but it can kill you if you hang onto it" (personal communication, 8 February 2018). He was telling me as bluntly but as kindly as he could that by sweating the stuff from the past, I would have health challenges in the present. I'm learning quickly to let go of the things I've grieved in the past because I care so much about my health and have the desire to live it long and well.

77. Life-saving universal law

I want to talk about another kind of balance: not the kind where you stand on one foot, put your finger on your nose, close your eyes, and try and walk in a straight line. No, this balance is big-picture balance, the universal law of balance that is so important to your wellbeing. Please bear with me as I explain this very important concept to you. It's a game- and life-changer!

Human behaviourist specialist Dr John Demartini draws on this philosophy in his work, which is a perfect blend of science and philosophy. Demartini (2018a) argues that in every event in our lives, we experience both sides (support and challenge) but often we are addicted to one side of life – predominantly seeking happiness. So when our happiness quotient doesn't measure up in our perception, we can tend towards depression because we're often hooked into a fantasy that everything should be positive and rosy. However, life isn't like that – every event has both sides – good and bad. Take, for example, going on a holiday, which we might perceive as something positive. However, there'll also be negative aspects to the holiday – perhaps you get a bad case of sunburn after lying on the beach for too long, or the people you holiday with might be real pains in the bottom, or eventually you get bored with the wonderful vacation, or its value didn't measure up to the cost, and so on. Alternatively, you could look at something you consider to be negative in your life – a tough upbringing for example. Just as the 'positive' holiday event outlined above also reveals negative aspects, there are positive aspects to something you perceive as negative. Perhaps you have developed greater independence now as a result of a 'rough childhood', that independence providing you with opportunities otherwise missed. Perhaps you are a very resilient person now and this has helped you in various areas of your life – vocational, personal, physical, etc. Maybe you went on to fill a void (something you have yearned to do) in your life that you wouldn't have filled had you not had that childhood experience. Once you can bring to mind or write down all the benefits of that childhood experience so that they equal emotionally those of the negative, then you can reach a place of gratitude and love for what is. And when you do that, you will experience fulfilment...until the next challenge comes along in your life, which invariably it will as the Universe is constantly conspiring for us to grow, and growth occurs at the border of support and challenge. Basically, there are no mistakes in life.

Demartini says that being addicted to only support and kindness (which makes us juvenile, dependent and obligated) will attract to us the opposites of challenge and unkindness (which make us independent and free) in order to break our addiction to support and kindness. So when you want too much of one aspect of life – positive, happy events – if this is out of balance, then your life will attract the opposite to bring you back into an equilibrated state (or balance). A perception of balance in our relationships is also important. Demartini believes that true love is the synthesis and synchronicity of complementary opposites – for example, the beautiful and the repulsive, the positive and negative, the good and bad, the happy and sad, the ups and downs of life in any relationship. You are in relationship to grow. Once you recognise the perfect balance (both positive and negative) that exists in everyone and everything around you and are grateful for the opportunities that this brings you, you are on the road to fulfilment.

This notion of synchronicity also relates to every moment in our lives. If you think on an event from the past in which you perceived someone doing something harmful to you, when you go back to that exact moment in your mind's eye and look for where you were supported by something/someone, you will find it if you are willing to see it! Try it again and again and each time you will find both sides (balance) operating in your life all of the time. It's quite wonderful to know that we are being challenged and supported in equal measure. There's an excellent 2016 film, *Collateral Beauty,* starring Will Smith and Helen Mirren, that addresses this philosophy in a powerful way. Smith's character, Howard Inlet, experiences a great tragedy causing him to retreat from life. The film explores how such a deep loss can also reveal moments of meaning and beauty. At a key moment in the film, Mirren, representing Death, says, "Don't forget to look for the collateral beauty", inviting the grief-stricken to see another side to the collateral damage associated with the trauma (IMDB, 2016). If you're challenged but intrigued by this topic, you might like to read Dr John Demartini's work for yourself for a more rewarding and fulfilled life. I recommend *The Breakthrough Experience: A Revolutionary New Approach to Personal Transformation* (2009), *The Gratitude Effect* (2008) and *The Values Factor: The Secret to Creating an Inspired and Fulfilling Life* (2013).

78. Vulnerability

Now there's a scary term! At least that's what I thought until I encountered Brene Brown through my research, an amazing woman who's a professor and vulnerability researcher at the University of Houston. Brown had been studying this topic for over 12 years by the time I read her work. You're probably wondering how being vulnerable could lead to a longer, healthier life. It's an indirect benefit actually. Vulnerability, according to Brown, is the feeling of "uncertainty, risk and emotional exposure". She cites an example to give us the picture: you turn up for your first-ever exercise class with your rubber mat and spandex wear, all set to transform your mind and body. But then you notice that all other students seem more confident striding into the studio, placing their mats with practised ease. You begin to withdraw, feel uncomfortable, less certain of your decision to turn up, your heart races, and you'd like to flee! This reaction is an example of vulnerability. When you don't run away, but rather stay in the heat, this is "vulnerability [at its] core, the heart, the center of meaningful experiences". Far from being a sign of weakness, these feelings of vulnerability are signs of great courage, according to Brown's research. She goes even further in arguing for vulnerability as the birthplace of emotions that we yearn for − expressions of "love, belonging, joy, courage, empathy, and creativity." Often, we might head for the exit door when we think no one is looking, considering ourselves unworthy and having feelings of I'm-just-not-good-enough bubbling to the surface of our minds. Hey, join the club − we've all been there. In the exercise class scenario above, we play a movie in our heads. It's no romantic comedy, but rather a blockbuster disaster film in which tragedy is the only outcome. Apart from losing out on the healing effects of this exercise class and the possibility of making new and interesting friends, the real tragedy is that in denying and negating this vulnerability, we're also missing out on love, belonging and joy!

Brown encourages us to "dare greatly". Daring greatly requires just a few steps. Firstly, you need to be mindful when next you experience this fragile moment of vulnerability. In that mindfulness you begin to face your emotions, recognising and acknowledging yourself for your courage in seeing it for what it is. Next, let go of the worry over what others think − you have no control over their thoughts anyway and it's likely they're going through their own stuff too. And finally, surrender to the notion of perfectionism − it doesn't exist. No one is perfect. Rather, just be the best example of who you are in that moment.

Practising vulnerability is a healing practice − healing the emotions. Emotional health is just as important as physical health. When you next experience feelings of "uncertainty, risk and emotional exposure", know that their opposites "love, belonging and joy" are waiting to reveal themselves in your vulnerability. A loving, connected and joyful spirit is certainly a recipe for good health in my book.

79. It's okay to say 'no'

I've had the privilege of working with many hundreds of women and men at personal development workshops over the years. They are courageous, powerful and inspiring people and they have taught me as much as if not more than I could ever impart to them. Yet, one theme seemed to stand out above many others: the inability to say no. I recognised the condition well, counting myself among their number. Too often we acquiesce to others, agreeing to things that we would rather say no to. Perhaps it's motivated by a desire to be liked and accepted, to please, to be friends; perhaps a fear of rejection. But you owe it to yourself to please *you* too. Whatever the reason, saying 'yes' when you mean 'no' may seem easier in the moment, but you pay the piper eventually, and it takes its toll on your emotional and physical health. You may be thinking that it's just too heartbreaking to say no to someone we care about. But when you think about it, saying yes when you mean no is insincere and those close to you deserve sincerity, don't you think? As do you. Human behaviourist, Dr John Demartini, has a powerful and cheeky philosophy in his book *The Breakthrough Experience* that's worked wonders for me when I'm caught between what I want to say and what I think others expect of me. He calls it the 'Law of Lesser Pissers' (Demartini, 2009) and believes "that if you're given the choice between pissing someone else off, or pissing yourself off, choose them. People come and go, but you're with you for the whole trip...and it's your life". When I first encountered this truism, it was a light-bulb moment: I'd never considered that inevitably *someone* in the exchange was going to be uncomfortable (pissed off) and that it didn't always need to be me. Once I accepted the truth of it, I felt liberated in giving more honest responses to others. Just one proviso: saying no doesn't mean you need to be rude. I believe if your truth is no, then you can deliver it honestly and with respect and gratitude to the other party. It may be that you simply need some time before deciding whether it's a yes or a no, so you could simply say, "Give me some time to think about it and I'll get back to you." If however, your body is screaming no, then you might say, "Thank you for the invitation but that's not the most appealing thing for me just now," or "Thank you but I don't have the time right now."

The other person may still be pissed off with what they perceive as rejection, but you've done it with respect and integrity. And besides, if they had respect for you, they'd respect your priorities.

If you have some strong personalities around you who may feel daunted at the prospect of their ideas or offers being declined, start small. Choose a salesperson or a telemarketer perhaps. With practice, saying no will become easier and you'll be better equipped to decline the more important interactions in your life (Gerst, 2017). If you aren't sure whether it's a yes or a no, then you'll need to become congruent with what is more important to you. See my discussion below, *Discover your purpose,* outlining the process determining your highest values so you know with certainty what you stand for.

There's an adage attributed to medical Doctor Gordon A Eadie: "stand for nothing, fall for anything" (1945). What he means is that if you don't have strong foundations (knowing your values), then you're likely to follow others aimlessly. Remember to stay true to yourself. If you're a chronic yes person, then your mental and physical health will suffer, and you'll eventually develop feelings of anger, resentment, despondency, and/or depression. Not a good state for a healthy mind and body, is it? Such negative emotions can foster anxiety and stress – and as you will have read elsewhere in this book, anxiety and stress correlate to disease in the body. So get out there and start practising some healthy, respectful and authentic noes.

80. Discover your purpose

Discovering why we're here and our true purpose in life is one of the most fulfilling things we can do, but it is often elusive to many of us. Aside from the intrinsic value we can bring to others, it's also significant for our own health and longevity. Studies have revealed that those who feel their lives have meaning and purpose are at a lower risk of heart disease and death. The Japanese call it *ikigai.* The Okinawans in Japan are heralded for their longevity, as healthy aging expert Professor Craig Wilcox (2001) discovered. Wilcox's study revealed that many of the Okinawan people have a sense of purpose. Could this be a reason so many of them exceed the 100-year mark? The concept of *ikigai* asks these questions: What do you love? What are you good at? What does the world need? What can you be paid for? The outcome of these questions is a greater sense of self-awareness which in turn leads to a more fulfilling life (Sigley, 2018). Over a seven-year period, 136,265 participants from across the United States and Japan were studied by Cohen, Bavishi and Rozanski. Those reporting a higher sense of purpose had around a 20% lower risk of death during that time. The researchers suggested that having a sense of purpose can shield us from stress responses and promote a healthier lifestyle, although they do concede they have not proven a cause and effect relationship between a sense of purpose and a longer life (Cohen, Bavishi & Rozanski, 2016). However, Dan Beuttner, in conjunction with National Geographic and a team of medical researchers, anthropologists, demographers, and epidemiologists, studied the longest-living people around the world and found that knowing one's purpose was one of nine key elements (the Power 9®) to health and longevity (2016).

So, how do we discover our higher purpose and live it? The best go-to person I know for this is Dr John Demartini. As a leading human behaviourist, Demartini says that our purpose is inherent and found in our highest values. The term *values* refers to the highest priorities in our lives. Our highest value is known as *telos* in ancient Greek, which translates as our chief aim and the study of meaning and purpose. Demartini argues that it's simply fear that blocks realising our purpose. But he has an inspiring solution: at the close of each day before sleep, he suggests getting a notepad and pen and reflecting on and writing down everything you are truly grateful for that day, until you experience a tear of gratitude. Then, turn inward into your most authentic and powerful self and ask these three questions: What message do you have for me today? What action steps am I to take to fulfil my life? What detail can you reveal about my life or mission? If you don't receive a message, just go back and reflect once more on what you can be truly grateful for, then ask the three questions again. You can repeat this process for a month or until you have clarity around your mission and purpose. All too often we look outside of ourselves for what we are meant to do. However, the wisdom lies within us. Demartini has a powerful mantra that has resonated in my life and I hope it does for you too: "When the voice and vision on the inside becomes louder and more profound than all the opinions on the outside, you have begun to master your life" (Demartini, 2017).

In conjunction with the gratitude and three-question process above is the practical and powerful 13-step method to determine your highest values and reveal your purpose in this life. It's known as the Demartini Value Determination & Application Process™, incorporating his Demartini Value Determination Process™ and the many variations of personal, professional and educational Demartini Value Application Processes™ (1989). Based on the study of axiology, an individual's unique hierarchy of human values determines how that individual will perceive and act upon the world. Human values are the foundation of human behaviour and the keys to development.

So, here's the process. Answer the following 13 questions, giving three examples of each – the three that are most important to you. Take some time to reflect on your answers and *be honest*. The only person who will benefit is *you*!

1. What do you fill your personal space (e.g. your home, your room, etc.) with?
2. How do you spend your time?
3. How do you spend your energy?
4. What do you spend your money on? (aside from any set expenses)
5. Where are you the most organised and ordered?
6. Where are you most disciplined and reliable?
7. What do you think about or focus on the most? (What dominates your thoughts?)
8. What do you envision (visualise) or dream about the most?
9. What do you most talk to yourself about (internal self-talk)?

10. What do you most often talk to others about?
11. What inspires you?
12. What goals stand out in your life and have stood the test of time?
13. What topics do you love to study, read about, or research?

You'll see you now have 39 answers to the 13 questions. There will be a certain amount of repetition – perhaps a lot! You may be expressing the same value in different ways, e.g. going out with my friends, eating with friends, etc. You will probably see a pattern begin to emerge. Look for the answer that is most often repeated and write the number 1 beside each same response. For example, if you wrote 'physical health, keeping fit, going to the gym, exercising', then put a number 1 beside each of those. Then look for the second most frequent answer and put a number 2 beside those. Then look for the third most frequent answer and put a number 3 beside those, and so on. Keep going until you feel you have given a number for each response. Now, create a list of your FIVE most important values in priority order, with the most important value first and the least important last:

1. _____
2. _____
3. _____
4. _____
5. _____

Now you have a firm foundation upon which to make decisions in your life. You can choose to say yes or no to any opportunities that come along and compare your decisions with your highest values. So, for example, if nutritional health is your number 1 value, then when faced with a choice between a burger and fries or a healthy alternative, it's a no-brainer which one you'll choose. Each time you choose to live by your highest values, you are on purpose. With the knowledge of your highest values, you've got the power and opportunity to shape your life, to ensure that your goals, your actions, your relationships, your career, and your highest values are aligned.

81. Become a lifelong learner

It makes sense, don't you think, that our brains are stimulated when we are constantly learning something new. When this happens, the learning process motivates the generation of new brain cells. Whether it's learning another language, playing word games, having a go at a new knitting pattern or craft, or putting yourself outside your comfort zone so that your brain does gymnastics, you're on a learning journey for a longer, healthier life.

I recently discovered that learning another language protects us against Alzheimer's. According to researchers at the York University in Toronto, for those who already have the disease but who are also bilingual, their brains function more efficiently and for several years longer than those who are monolingual (Craik, Bailystok & Freedman, 2010).

I began knitting again after about a 30-year gap. My first serious sojourn into the knitting world manifested as a woollen cardigan for my betrothed – a complex weave of cabling, slipping, casting, and swearing, among many other mind-altering challenges. Sadly, he didn't wear it often because the wool made him itchy and our subtropical Queensland climate wasn't conducive to frequent wool wearing. However, in time, I returned to the craft with the help of a friend and now I'm knitting a cotton blanket for my granddaughter. It's made up of little squares and some complex patterning. As I'm in the infant stages of the blanket, my concentration levels are high, and I can almost hear the rust scraping away from the internal cogs of my brain as I try to master this craft again. Knitting is said to be as therapeutic as yoga and distracts from chronic pain, lowers blood pressure, reduces depression, and may even be attributable to slowing the onset of dementia (Knapton, 2018) – swearing aside, of course, when I've dropped a stitch! Just to give knitting one more rap, Albert Einstein is said to have knitted to "calm his mind and clear his thinking" (Clark et al, 2015). Perhaps it helped him unravel the mysteries of $E=MC^2$.

If you want to become a real brain junkie, I'd recommend computerised brain games, be they digital photography, Photoshop, word games, mathematical games, a new digital game that tests the grey matter, or whatever takes your fancy as long as it stretches you mentally. I've tried Lumosity which is a brilliant and fun app for developing your brain through science games. The app is free but for a small fee you can purchase a more comprehensive brain-training version. While being active in any field of your choice is wonderful for good brain health, ultimately the message here is that it's the learning of a *new skill* that has the most profound and significant gains on your mental acuity (Park *et al*, 2014: 103-12).

82. Invest in a mentor or life coach

The seventeenth-century English author, John Donne, once wrote that, "No man is an island of itself; every man is a piece of the continent, a part of the main; if a clod be washed away by the sea, Europe is the less, as well as if a promontory were, as well as any manner of thy friends or of thine own were; any man's death diminishes me, because I am involved in mankind. And therefore never send to know for whom the bell tolls; it tolls for thee." Gender-specific language aside, Donne's observation is as relevant today as it was then. What I believe Donne is saying is that none of us is totally self-reliant, each being dependent on the other, that we're all connected and that the death of anyone diminishes us all.

I'd like to link Donne's sentiment to our twenty-first century context and the wellbeing that can be derived from seeking guidance and wisdom from others. The term 'life coaching' is a relatively recent one, arising in the 1980s, but the notion of a mentor first emerged in Homer's Odyssey (around 850BC) when Odysseus, King of Ithaca, travelled away from his home for some 10 years. During his long sojourn, a mentor was entrusted with the care of Odysseus' household and in particular, his son, Telemachus.

In time, the term 'mentor' came to mean a trusted advisor, friend, teacher, and wise person. Gordon Shea (1997) describes the field of mentoring as a basic form of human development where one individual invests their "time, energy and personal know-how in assisting the growth and ability of another person". Mentoring and life coaching have become synonymous, with both roles designed to guide and inspire us to succeed in our personal and/or professional lives, especially when we find we are not achieving on our own. I'll use the term 'mentor' for the remainder of this topic with the understanding that the term 'life coach' is also inferred.

While a therapist or counsellor is primarily skilled at exploring a client's past traumas that negatively affect their lives, a mentor generally works with people who are looking to the future and seeking more success or better relationships, realising a vision, and so on. They're a 'guide-on-the-side', keeping you accountable (perhaps for achieving your goals) and helping you accomplish what you cannot do on your own. An effective mentor won't offer advice as such, but they'll listen to you, ask incisive questions and challenge you, all to support the changes you wish to experience in your life.

The 'challenge' element is the most powerful component to a mentor's role. John Demartini argues that the greatest growth (innovation, creation and opportunity) you will experience is at the border of support and challenge, which a wise and powerful mentor can facilitate (Demartini, 2015). There are many examples of successful mentor–student relationships. The ancient Greek philosopher, Plato, was mentored by Socrates. Plato went on to become the pre-eminent philosopher in our Western tradition. In our modern era we have figures such as Oprah Winfrey whose mentor was the celebrated author and poet, the late Maya Angelou. Mark Zuckerberg, Facebook's CEO, was mentored by Apple Inc. founder, the late Steve Jobs. Nobel-prize-winning Mother Teresa, the Catholic nun who dedicated her life to the poor and dying of Calcutta, was mentored by Father Michael van der Peet (Rhodes, 2015). While each of these has realised amazing achievements in their lives, which we might assume can (in part at least) be attributed to the wisdom and guidance of those who mentored them, there are many thousands of 'ordinary' folk who've gone on to be the best versions of themselves through the benefits of mentoring.

Dr John Demartini has mentored thousands of people in his role as a human behaviourist. He compares the frustration of trying to do something on your own through trial and error (akin to banging your head against a wall) to the wisdom that comes from a mentor, using a twelfth-century metaphor 'standing on the shoulders of giants' (Demartini, 2017), which means to discover truth by building on previous discoveries. By drawing on the understanding gained by others who have gone before us, we make personal and professional progress in our lives. Through mentorship, we build on their strengths and are enhanced as human beings in whatever field we are exploring. The alternative, reinventing the wheel through trial and error, is a slow and potentially painful process.

There are two important caveats to the role of mentor. Firstly, they are there to provide wisdom and guidance, but it is not about becoming them, rather, it's about learning from them, then shaping what you've learned to suit your own unique circumstances. Secondly, it's important to choose a mentor who recognises and values what is important to you and who shapes their guidance with this in mind. Or better still, someone whose values align with yours (Demartini, 2017). When you are being your authentic self and developing your skills, talents and abilities with the help of others, you are giving expression to a fuller life.

So how does working with a mentor help us gain better health and thus, a longer life? To answer this question I'll simply say that we don't know what we don't know! Sometimes we need others to help us see and do what we have become consciously or subconsciously blinded to. For instance, you may be highly stressed at work. You have been doing this routine for years. It's become habitual. You don't like it, but you don't know why, and you can't seem to navigate a way out of the mire. However, the wisdom within you knows that you're not an island (as Donne says), so seeking out a wise mentor can help steer you through those muddied waters.

As I've mentioned elsewhere in this book, stress can be a killer, or at the very least, detrimental to your health. Stress can lead to the pH in your body becoming more acidic, and an acidic state can be an unhealthy disease-inducing state. Also, the aging process can be accelerated when you are under prolonged stress. Muscular pain can also often develop, and the stress response is said to stimulate cortisol which increases insulin levels and thus inflammation (Hyman, nd). If prolonged or ongoing stress is your experience, then a mentor to help you see another way of being and improve your health along the way is a worthy consideration. A wise mentor will consider not just your emotional state to bring you into balance. They'll consider you holistically, encompassing all areas of your life – emotional, physical, behavioural, nutritional, financial, spiritual, vocational, and familial. They will help you set meaningful goals across all areas of your life so that it would be impossible not to make giant leaps in your wellbeing. I recently read Turia Pitt's book *Unmasked,* which I've mentioned elsewhere under the heading of *An attitude of gratitude*, but I'd like to repeat her story here because it's so powerful. She would have to be one of the most inspirational and goal-driven human beings I've ever encountered. In 2011, she was competing in an ultramarathon in Western Australia's Kimberley region when she was caught in a bushfire, suffering burns to 64% of her body. From near-death and against all odds, she eventually went on to do some amazing physically and mentally challenging events, including two Ironman events in Port Macquarie (Australia) and Kona (Hawaii). In discussing the right mindset for achieving whatever we might want to achieve, Pitt tells us we need to "get comfortable being uncomfortable" (Pitt & Corbett, 2018, p.257), stepping outside our comfort zone and setting "stretch goals". Motivational speaker Charlie 'Tremendous' Jones talked of the power of outside influences when he said, "You will be the same person in five years as you are today except for the people you meet and the books you read" (Tremendous Leadership, 2018). Pitt has been that outside influence for many people since the 2011 bushfire.

When you set SMARTT goals (**S**pecific, **M**easurable, **A**chievable, **R**elevant, **T**argeted, and **T**imed) that are aligned with your highest values and designed to serve others, you are increasing the probability of having a fulfilled life. Filling your day with high-priority actions and delegating low-priority activities to others is inspirational. "Nobody gets up in the morning and dedicates their life to your dreams. Your dreams are up to you" (Demartini, 2016). Those dreams can be made real with the support of a mentor. If you recognise that the person you are today isn't the person you wish to become, then seek outside guidance through a mentor. They'll help you live a purpose-filled life. As I wrote under the topic *Discover your purpose*, statistics show that participants with a purpose are more likely to have a lower risk of heart disease and a 20% lower risk of death compared to those who do not identify their purpose (Cohen, Bavishi & Rozanski, 2016). Based on my own experiences and the findings of giants whose shoulders I've attempted to stand on, it would seem that a mentor is a good investment for your life.

83. Saving and tracking spending

You're probably wondering how saving and tracking your spending could possibly lead to future-proofing your health. I hope I will have made the connection for you by the close of this topic. About seven years ago, I attended a seminar facilitated by Dr John Demartini. One key aspect of that event centred on financial freedom and wealth. A take-home message for me was the power in beginning to save a portion of my money each month, the idea being that that money would then start working for me, so I could eventually raise my lifestyle. I was soon to find out just how powerful that process would be. At the time of the seminar I was fairly adept at *spending* money, but I wasn't so great at the other end of the spectrum: *saving*. Demartini told us that while we might believe we value money our lives often demonstrate the opposite. A depleted bank balance and elevated credit card debt are usually good clues to a lack of appreciation of the value of money. At time of writing, Australians have clocked up a $32.6 billion credit card debt, an average of $4,200 per cardholder (ASIC, 2018). That converts to a lot of accumulated stress! The key, according to Demartini, is valuing money in order to save it (Demartini, personal communication, 29 November 2011).

Aside from the practical process of setting aside a portion of your income each month, a good way to begin is by reading and learning about finances and money management. Two books he recommended are *The Richest Man in Babylon* by George S Clason and *How to Make One Hell of a Profit and Still Get to Heaven* by John Demartini. At the time, without undertaking any reading on the subject or increasing my income, I set up an automatic electronic transfer of funds to an account I creatively called 'Savings Account'. Initially, I transferred just $100 a month to this account. Over time, I have systematically increased the monthly amount and watched my savings grow exponentially. I didn't consciously cut back on spending and I didn't receive any special windfalls, but there was definite power simply in starting the process of saving and persisting with it. At some subconscious level though, I must have been cutting back on unnecessary expenses for the money to grow to the level it has. Another key ingredient to this process, as suggested by Demartini, is having an attitude of gratitude for our savings. 'Money flows where gratitude grows' is the mindset, the idea being that appreciating and being grateful for the savings in your account will lead to more savings.

You might now be thinking, Great, looks simple, let's get started. Or perhaps you're questioning the viability of such an approach or dismissing the notion altogether. You're probably right to be a little circumspect for there *is* another element to this process that's just as significant for the savings 'magic' to work. It's called service. We need to give (service) and receive (reward) in equal measure. It is a form of exchange, if you will, rather than just passively waiting for financial gain to come whizzing to our front door. Sadly, it will whizz by if you aren't doing both. Demartini argues that the reason we have been given both sensory and motor functions is that we're here on the planet to undertake service with our motor functions and to receive reward with our sensory functions. If you are operating in a fair exchange mode, then there is no limit to what you can save (Hendry, 2018). With all this in mind, there are 10 practical habits you can follow to remain debt-free and build your savings. Following these, according to Demartini, fosters an inspired life within your means and allows you to gradually expand those means. This, in turn, allows you to live a richer and more fulfilled life (Demartini, 2017a). These 10 healthy savings habits are outlined below:

- Monitor your personal finances, pay attention to details, budget, and make sure you do not waste your money
- Research, learn and govern your finances – know what your essential costs are
- Pretend you make less and live within your means to increase your savings
- Think wisely and long-term, rather than foolishly and impulsively for immediate gratification
- Be willing to ask for more reasonable deals or interest rates – ask and you shall receive
- Habitually and electronically save ever-greater portions of your income
- Set specific long-term goals worth saving and investing for
- Say no to spending temptations and non-priority expenses that might enslave you
- Value using cash to keep yourself aware of your actual expenses
- Value experiences and any investments that will appreciate in value over simply accumulating transient/short-term consumables and depreciable items.

With reference to Demartini's first point, I've recently learned of a free Aussie-inspired app called 'TrackMySpend' to record your personal expenses. The app categorises your expenses and you can set it to limit your spend per week within categories. It's worth checking out if you're interested in curbing your spending and saving more.

I've already mentioned above how saving, serving and tracking spending can inspire you to live a more fulfilled life, but did you know there are other health benefits to saving your dollars? Having a nest egg of savings can reduce your stress levels. Living from one pay packet to the next without reserves can be harrowing. Conflicts in relationships often revolve around money concerns, causing unnecessary distress for all parties involved. Health conditions such as anxiety, depression, insomnia, and more serious illnesses are often a follow-on from stresses triggered by money worries (Gupta, 2016). Having cash reserves can relieve that anxiety and reduce the consequent risk of ill-health, should you ever experience an unexpected and costly event.

Many of the health topics I've written about elsewhere in this book will also save you money: quitting smoking, reducing your alcohol consumption, walking or cycling instead of driving, eating a Mediterranean diet rather than processed food... What it all comes down to is: if your intention is to make your century hale and hearty, then you'll obviously need the funds to enjoy that extended life as well. Money may not ensure happiness but if treated with respect and gratitude, it can provide you with a means to better health.

84. Love and kindness

Where would we all be without a drop of human love and kindness in our lives? This is an important topic and one that I may not do justice to in the confines of these pages, but if I did not include it, it would leave my philosophy about health and longevity lacking. I'm reminded of that fabulous film released in 2000, *Pay It Forward*, where seventh-grader Trevor McKinney takes on a social studies assignment to change the world for the better. His philosophy is simple: when someone does you a favour or shows you a kindness, rather than returning it, 'pay it forward' to three people who would not otherwise be able to do this thing for themselves. They, in turn, do the same and so the practice of helping others spreads within society and, presumably, across the globe. This little boy initiates a social movement to make the world a better place (IMDB, 2000). Love drives the movement.

I'm not talking about romantic, infatuated, love here, but love that is at the essence of our being, that is ever-present and intuitively guiding us at all times (Demartini, 2015). Human behaviourist Dr John Demartini (2013: 163) defines love as the synthesis and synchronicity of all complementary opposites in the Universe.

In other words, whenever something is challenging you in your life, there's also something supporting you; whenever someone is accepting you, there's another rejecting you, and so on. At the intersection of these seemingly opposing forces is love. This universal law of balance is ever-present across all aspects of our lives. William Shakespeare, the greatest writer in the English language, recognised and wrote of life's symmetry of opposites when he penned "the web of life is of a mingled yarn, good and ill together" (*All's Well That Ends Well*, IV, 3, 80). Embracing both sides of life is a truly balanced perception of life. As I've just mentioned, at the intersection of these opposing forces (challenge/support, acceptance/rejection, good/bad and so on) resides love.

While I've used a fictional example to open this topic, there's lots of real-world evidence where love is expressed for the betterment of humanity. The 1989 Tiananmen Square incident comes to mind and reflects Demartini's understanding of love. An unidentified man is filmed while he stands in front of a line of tanks on 5 June that year in response to the Chinese military's violent suppression of the Tiananmen Square protestors. This David and Goliath, man-versus-tank standoff, is an example of love (*and* courage*)* and represents a powerful force for the betterment of humankind. According to political scientist and historian, Benjamin Barth (2014), the event ceased the Chinese occupation of Tiananmen Square and pointed to more hopeful signs of China's "liberal concepts based on constitutionalism and democratic participation". That's big-picture stuff, I know, and perhaps you might find it somewhat challenging to see love in both what we perceive to be 'bad' as well as 'good'!

Anthony Robbins alludes to this dichotomy by posing a telling question when faced with challenges in our lives: What would love do right now? Robbins recognises that letting love lead the way in the face of challenges benefits not only others, but also ourselves (2012). There are so many 'little' incidents of love around us that make for a better world and a better us, ones that don't require standing in front of an armoured vehicle for evidence of love's efficacy. "Love is the eternal, trans-dimensional quantum field of creation and communication that all forms of life arise out of and are inexorably joined by. We are created by small expressions of Love, yet our greatest potential for creation and communication depend on our ability to channel as much Love as possible" (Kopecky, 2016).

We see these 'small expressions of love' everywhere we care to look. A mother tends a screaming child in the busy aisles of a supermarket; cars stop on a fast-paced highway to make way for a family of ducks; an Australian man gives out hugs in 2004 leading to a global hug campaign; we get up each day and go to work, look after our family, visit a sick friend, and so on. These random acts of kindness and commitment, when selfless, make others feel better. And when we are faced with the opposing force – hate – Brene Brown (2015) suggests we "move in closer" rather than be repelled by others. It's hard to hate someone close up, Brown concludes. When we get to know someone, we discover they're more than just their political affiliations, their class, their sexual orientation, and so on. They're human beings with vulnerabilities and strengths like the rest of us. Then, of course, there's the most important person we need to love, and that is ourself. How can we love others if we don't love ourselves – not in an egotistical sense, but one that is balanced and inclusive? Loving ourself, not because of our faults, but in spite of them.

Love may choose to play hardball too; it's known as 'tough love'. For example, a parent denies a drug-addicted child financial support until she enters drug rehabilitation. Bill Milliken coined the phrase *tough love* back in 1968 in his co-authored book by that name (Milliken & Meredith, 1968). The term refers to treating someone seemingly harshly but with the intention of helping them in the long run. It is love that motivates and drives the toughness.

Now, the good news for your longevity is that genuine expressions of love are good for your physical and emotional health. Love positively intensifies your mood, which is triggered by increased dopamine levels in the brain. Love reduces your stress levels, eases anxiety and helps you to live longer because of the connection to others that it creates (Ducharme, 2018). When you look for opportunities to practise kind and loving acts, you are doing yourself and others a great service. As Max Erhmann wrote, "In the face of all aridity and disenchantment [love] is as perennial as the grass" (1927). I'll leave it to the ascetic and sage, the Buddha, to conclude this topic. He taught that "none of the means employed...has a sixteenth part of the value of loving-kindness. Loving-kindness, which is freedom of the heart, absorbs them all; it glows, it shines, it blazes forth" (Kopecky, 2016).

85. Sex and intimacy

You're probably thinking that when you're in the mood for or engaging in sex, one of your highest priorities may *not* be how this activity might boost your immune system, reduce your weight and extend your life! Sex is meant to be a pleasurable experience and that in itself may be the only reason you need to indulge. However, since my researcher's brain has had me exploring everything from proper pooping positions to the merits of dental flossing, I couldn't let this important topic go unexplored, especially if having regular sex meant enjoying a longer and livelier life.

I was pleasantly surprised to discover the benefits are many and manifold. For instance, did you know that having sex boosts your libido? Dr Lauren Streicher (2017) says that for women it increases the vaginal fluids, blood flow and elasticity of the vagina, which heighten your feelings of wellbeing and make you crave more. On a more mundane level but no less important it is said to develop the pelvic floor muscles, which leads to greater bladder control. While acknowledging that masturbation also has an important part to play in our sex lives, sexual intercourse, as opposed to masturbation, lowers your systolic blood pressure (the first number on your blood pressure reading). The Duke Medical Center in North Carolina undertook a women's study, which determined that a history of a healthy and active sex life was one of the top three most significant indicators for enhanced longevity (Glasson, 2014). It's great exercise too, burning about five calories per minute. Every calorie counts! There's a lower risk of heart attack due to the greater balance in oestrogen and testosterone levels. Prostate cancer is said to be less likely, with more frequent ejaculation. Orgasm is said to be a brilliant pain blocker, releasing a hormone that lifts your pain threshold, and vaginal stimulation is said to reduce menstrual cramping, arthritic pain and even headaches (Komisaruk, 2017). Sex also releases stress and improves sleep. But above all, it is an opportunity for intimacy and closeness which is a powerful potion for living a longer and healthier life.

If you wanted evidence for the benefits of sexual activity to your health and longevity, then you need look no further than the Italian town of Acciaroli where 81 of the 700 residents there have passed their century. Researchers from San Diego's School of Medicine spent six months studying these older residents' lifestyles and learned (I'm not sure how) of their 'rampant' sex lives. They also have excellent blood circulation, equivalent to what you'd find in people in their 20s and 30s (Cockburn, 2016). So perhaps sex is an elixir for long life. French author, Marie de Hennezel, writes of aging and intimacy in her book *Sex After Sixty* (2017). de Hennezel recognises that as we age, the flame of sexual intimacy does not need to go out but in fact can become more emotional and erotic. However, we do need to work on it. She relays a sexual therapist's philosophy of the importance of getting to know each other by spending time looking at each other, talking about feelings and then having a physical connection such as a hug, a real hug, as a space for sexual intimacy to be nurtured. In addition to de Hennezel's work, if you'd like to read more about how to develop a more sensual, sexual and satisfying sex life, then Australia's leading sex expert, Dr Rosie King, has a fabulous book titled *Good Loving Great Sex* (2011). And if you're looking to learn more about the link between sexuality, happiness and wellbeing, then Jacqueline Hellyer of The LoveLife Clinic in Sydney is worth researching. Hellyer is a certified psychosexual therapist who helps individuals and couples develop greater awareness and confidence around sex, love and intimacy. Her clinic is also lesbian, bisexual, gay, transgender, queer, intersexual, and asexual (LBGTQIA) positive, welcoming clients of all sexual orientations. Sex may not always be seamless: it means becoming vulnerable, revealing yourself physically, emotionally and/or psychologically. It may mean some awkward fumbling and experimentation, exploring new realms with your sexual partner. And that's all absolutely okay. So, what are you waiting for? Give your partner that 'come hither' look when you see them next, knowing that it's not only a pleasurable pastime but one that's good for your life, your libido and your longevity.

86. Fun and laughter truly are the best medicine

The phrase 'laughter is the best medicine' is obscure in its origins but may be attributed to twentieth-century American humourist and publisher, Bennett Cerf, although some suggest it goes back a little further, being derived from Proverbs 17:22 which says that "a merry heart is like medicine". The meaning however is clear: laughter is said to be a cure for physical and emotional ailments (Lighthouse, 2016). This is no idle interpretation, but one based on scientific research. A 15-year Norwegian study of 53,556 participants was released in 2016 revealing that people with a sense of humour outlive those who don't laugh as much (Romundstad *et al*, 2016: 345-353). When we were children, laughter usually came to us spontaneously and often. As adults, it's time to reclaim that humour because it will not only make us feel good, but it is incredibly beneficial to our physical, emotional and social health.

Robinson, Smith & Segal (2017) outline a number of life-giving benefits to laughter that are backed by scientific evidence. Robinson *et al* argue that laughter relaxes your muscles, dissipating tension; boosts the immune system; releases the happy hormones (endorphins); protects the heart through increased blood flow; and burns calories. If you laugh for up to 15 minutes a day, you'll burn 40 calories equating to almost two kg a year. You'll also be lightening any heavy load you might be carrying emotionally: humour can diffuse conflict and help you see the lighter side of a problem. And, of course, this all equates to a longer life, as the Norwegian study attests. Robinson and his associates (2017) also say that laughter and humour can strengthen relationships, make us more attractive to others, improve teamwork, and promote group bonding.

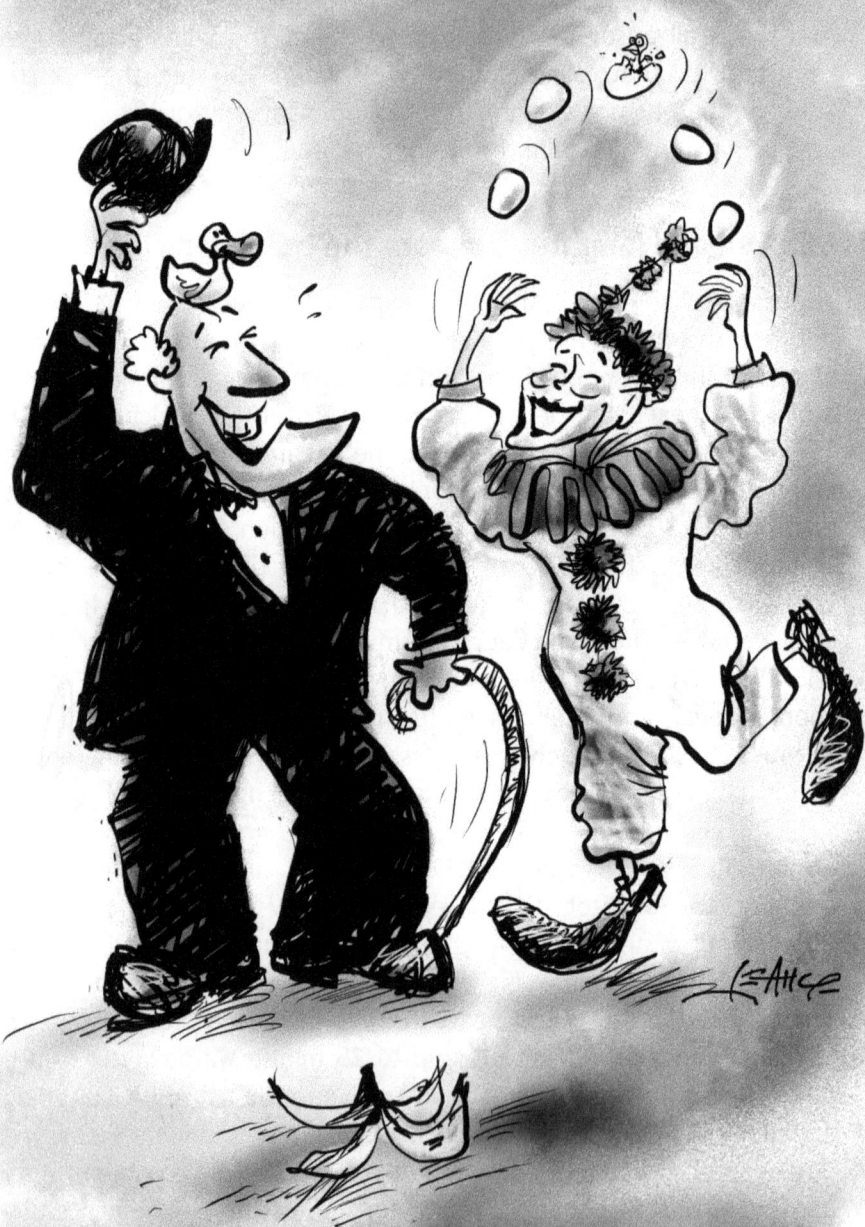

There are a number of ways you can bring genuine laughter into your life. Spending time with fun and playful people is always a good start. Going to a good comedy routine is always sure to elicit a good belly laugh. Bringing humour into your conversations is another way: for instance, at the end of your day when you might be sitting around the dinner table with your family/friends, why not ask them about the funniest thing that happened that day? (Robinson *et al,* 2017). Australian comedian, Julia Morris, has had her fair share of challenges and chuckles in her life. There's one constant that's helped her overcome all sorts of hurdles in her life: finding humour in the everyday. Morris tells us: "I often think about the great catchphrase of people looking for the perfect work-life balance and I'm telling you, it doesn't exist. What you actually need to look for is the laughs in each day. That's what keeps you buoyant" (King, 2017).

If you want evidence of the health and longevity benefits of joy and laughter, take another look at Japanese doctor Shigeaki Hinohara who lived to 105. Hinohara said that one of his secrets to a long life was a fervent belief in having fun. He was also a great advocate for not losing our childlike joy of the world as we enter adulthood (Gillett, 2017). While there are many well-meaning organisations designed to bring people together specifically for collective laughter as a tonic, I'm more of an advocate for spontaneous feelings of joy and outbursts of laughter as tonics for greater health and wellbeing.

87. Music to save your life and build your happiness quotient

Music is medicine. After doing some research into the therapeutic benefits of music and good health, I had a little chuckle to myself. Google revealed a number of interesting sites – the first one stating '5 ways music can help you stay healthy', then '8 amazing health benefits of music', and then '15 amazing benefits of listening to music…' It didn't take me long to recognise that all the sites I surfed had the same underlying themes, which I'll summarise as 'five key ways music can keep you happy and healthy'. Perhaps unsurprisingly, the main benefit of listening to music is reducing anxiety, whether you're tuned into the dulcet tones of Celine Dion, or Deep Purple's heavy metal amplifications. If you're in a foul mood or feeling overwhelmed and stressed, music is your medicine. Heavy metal music is said to have a cathartic effect on anger, so says a study from the University of Queensland (Sharman & Dingle, 2015). And of course, relaxing music is an excellent way to help you pack up all your cares and woes. As eighteenth-century English playwright, Willian Congreve, so eloquently put it, "Musick has charms to soothe a savage breast."

Secondly, music is great for helping you sleep. According to music therapist Dr Amy Clements-Cortes (Lee & Clements-Cortes, 2014), there is an effective trend towards using music to facilitate sleep and relaxation, and even if you listen to music earlier in the day, you'll still reap the rewards of a good night's sleep later.

Next, there's the boost to your immune system which is so important in safeguarding against disease and illness. A study undertaken at Pennsylvania's Wilkes University reveals that the background music you hear in a lift or when you're on hold on the telephone – more commonly referred to as 'muzak' – elevates a vital antibody known as immunoglobulin A (IgA) (Charnetski, Brennan & Harrison, 1998). This study compared other tested groups who were subject to the more mundane tone click or radio program. The muzak group had markedly increased levels of IgA. Another benefit to the soothing tones elicited by music is that it is said to reduce pain. A study undertaken by the University of Granada in 2016 on patients with the debilitating disease fibromyalgia, characterised by chronic musculoskeletal pain, found that when patients listened to music in conjunction with guided imagery, they experienced reduced stress, a lessening in their pain and a greater sense of wellbeing. Aside from the obvious health benefits here, the researchers acknowledged the cost-effectiveness and ease of implementing such a treatment (Andre, 2016).

Dr Shigeaki Hinohara promoted music therapy at St Luke's Hospital for his patients, with positive results. The music was said to help the

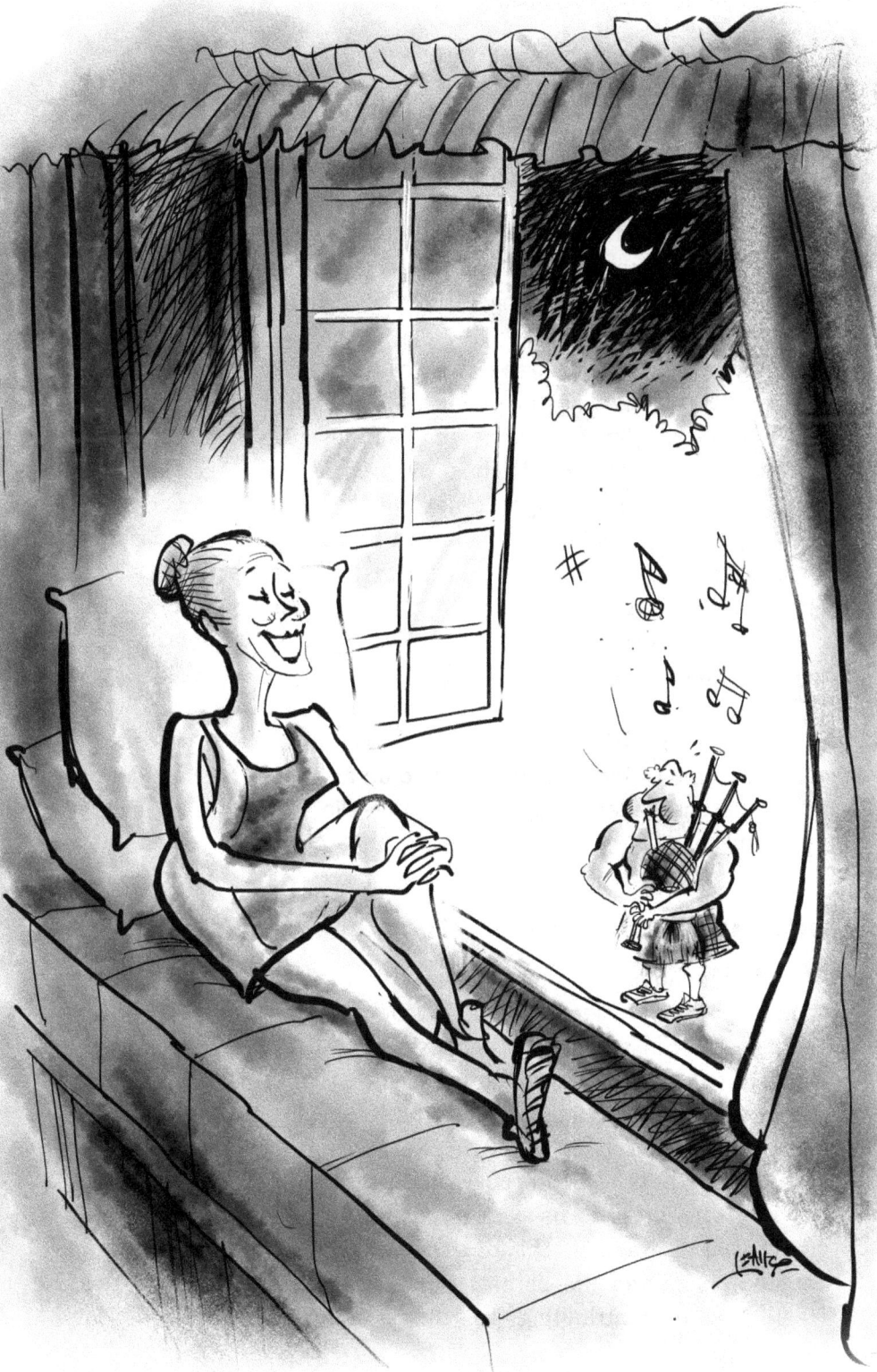

patients gain physical and emotional wellbeing and healing (Gillett, 2017). Delta Goodrem, Australian singer and songwriter, has had her own battles with chronic ill-health, having been diagnosed with Hodgkin's lymphoma when she was just 18. Now in her 30s and in great physical and mental health, she acknowledged that music has been her best medicine. "Music's been an incredible healer for me over the years," she says (King, 2017).

And finally, music can act as a weight-loss program! Yes folks, if you need to lose a few kilos or pounds, all you might need to do is sit back, relax and listen to some gentle tunes such as a soft jazz to reduce your weight. Researchers Wansink & Van Ittersum (2012) undertook a study through Cornell University and discovered that soft lighting and gentle music equated to less food being consumed and a greater enjoyment of the meal into the bargain. So your physiology is positively impacted by music, causing you to eat less. A smaller waistline is a plus when you're looking to improve your health and wellbeing.

To end this tip, let's leave it to 1970's singer and songwriter, Eric Carmen, who crooned, 'Turn the radio up for that sweet sound, Hold me close, never let me go, Keep this feelin' alive.' Feeling *alive* is what this book is all about!

88. Multigenerational and community connection

This topic addresses family connection as well as the social connections of friendships and community. The opposite of connection can often be loneliness. In a 2015 meta-analysis on loneliness, researchers identified that social isolation, whether perceived or actual, increased the odds of dying by an astounding 45% (Holt-Lunstsad *et al*, 2015). Researchers in longevity, Lynda Grattan and Andrew Scott (2016), believe that a key to living a long and healthy life is to have closer bonds and connection with our families. For example, children spending time with grandparents not only supports the parents but also helps the older relatives feel they're contributing to their grandchildren's lives. The grandchildren experience a broader support and connection with family beyond their parents. Often, in our current social and cultural circumstances, together with the tyranny of distance between families, there is an "institutional [and] spatial segregation" that occurs between generations of families (Grattan & Scott, 2016). This can set up an 'us' and 'them' mindset, which in turn can lead to feelings of isolation and rejection – a state ripe for ill-health. Once upon a time, families of different ages lived closer, fostering more face-to-face interactions. And while we might attempt to visit our relatives and friends periodically, Grattan & Scott argue for a more sustained familiarity that leads to longer, healthier lives. What that means is having "stable, lasting interactions over time". If this is not always possible, then the researchers acknowledge that friendships across age groups also have a positive impact on diminishing the social segregation of the young and old. Professor Perminder Sachdev, head of the Sydney Centenarian Study, argues that it is the "quality of your social network and your relationships... that matters. It is part of your happiness now, but also for your long and happy life" (Edmistone, 2017). Centenarian Katharine Weber, who celebrated her last birthday at the age of 108, knew the value of connection to longevity: she faithfully made the Sunday roast with her family each week. One of her two sons, Thomas, speaking in 2014, said that those "Sunday dinners are a tradition we're never going to give up" (Glasson, 2014).

Gratton (2016) asks her students to project themselves into their older years, having them consider what advice they would give their older selves. Their responses include the importance of building friendships. Grattan agrees, arguing that not enough time is devoted to developing lasting career and personal friendships to keep our brains functioning well and the chance to keep learning. In our twenty-first century, we can stay connected with family and friends across the globe through social media and a range of digital technologies. At the heart of these philosophies is a truism: the need for connection and communication between human beings within and across the generations. The outcome leads to not only a healthier, longer-living you, but a more connected community of people.

89. Volunteering and contributing lengthens your life

Ancient Greek philosopher Aristotle once asked and answered the following: "What is the essence of life? To serve others and do good." Giving up your time for others has benefits beyond the altruistic feel-good component. If you've ever helped out at a charity event, or assisted on a stall at a school fete, or simply given a half-hour of your time at any community event through a sense of service rather than self-gratification, then you'll understand this feel-good notion. It's otherwise known as the "helper's high" (Baraz & Alexander, 2010).

You'll be pleased to learn that you are also being rewarded with good *physical* health too. In a study conducted in 2013 by Carnegie Mellon University, volunteers aged over 50 experienced lower blood pressure, thereby reducing their risk of heart disease, stroke and premature death. Consistency and regularity of service seems to be the key here though. In the Carnegie Mellon study, participants who contributed 200 hours per year to volunteering for the right reasons experienced lower blood pressure. The study also revealed that volunteer work was often associated with stress reduction, a factor that is strongly linked to positive health outcomes (Watson, 2013). Besides, giving your time to others is also a great way to meet new people, thereby broadening your social connections and perhaps learning something new into the bargain. While the correlation between volunteering and lowered blood pressure among the participants in the above study cannot be interpreted as absolute proof, other studies have revealed similar findings (Watson, 2013). I came across the fantastic example of Dr Shigeaki Hinohara, who I mention several times in this book. Hinohara was a physician, chairman emeritus of St Luke's International University and an honorary president of St Luke's International Hospital. He recommended several tenets for a long and healthy life. Among them, he believed that life was all about contributing. He had an amazing drive to help people, so he would wake early each morning and do something good for others. He would set goals around how he could help people and until a few months before his death on 18 July 2017, Hinohara was still treating patients and making a contribution (Gillett, 2017).

Suffice to say, we're helping ourselves and others in our community by volunteering and other contributions. A win-win, wouldn't you say? I've enjoyed about five years of volunteering at a local animal shelter and I look forward to my four-hour shift each week. It is rewarding playing a small part in bringing pets and their new families together. Doing some good in serving others might just be the essence of a healthy life, as our ancient friend Aristotle reasoned.

90. Embrace and capitalise on your age

The idea of growing older might frighten or even repel many of us (not that we can escape it!). If we look outside of ourselves at the cultural perception of aging, there seems to be a pervading stereotype of the 'older generation' as having "shakier handwriting, poorer memories, higher rates of cardiac disease and lower odds of recovering from disability" among other age-related phenomena (Tergesen, 2015). It would seem that these conditions are exacerbated by an entrenched *negative* belief around aging. However, something marvellous occurs when we perceive our advancing years as a place of *opportunity* and *growth*: our self-image, strength and balance are said to improve; we can add an extra seven and a half years to our life expectancy compared with those who see aging as undesirable; our relationships are said to be enhanced; and a positive perception around aging can also improve our memory.

My women readers might be familiar with the archetype of the Great Goddess as maiden, mother and crone. The latter term has, in the past, held disturbing connotations but psychiatrist and Jungian analyst, Dr Jean Bolen, is helping to make a shift towards a different notion of crone in what she describes as the "juicy crone" phase – seeing the crone years as a crowning glory in one's life (2014). It's a time, Bolen argues, where you experience greater authenticity, you can use your life's wisdom to make a real difference in the world. Interestingly, younger women are actually looking for a wise elder as role models. They're wanting to know what's possible in the last third of their lives. As Bolen states, "Something is stirring in us that wants to be alive, that wants to be a source of inspiration and information" (2014).

Dr Libby Weaver also has an encouraging philosophy around age. With age, Weaver argues, come experience, wisdom, greater spiritual awareness, and emotional maturity (2013: 11). What a wonderful 'load' to bear. As Max Ehrmann (1952) wrote in *Desiderata*: "Take kindly the counsel of the years, gracefully surrendering the things of youth." Sixty-year-old social media star and model, Sarah Jane Adams, has moved beyond surrender of youth to a real embrace of her age (Hooper, 2017). On Adams' Instagram page, @mywrinklesaremystripes, she draws a parallel with her wrinkles which she wears with pride, arguing that "in the military, stripes are an accolade, a mark of commendation." Good on you, Sarah! I believe that younger women (and men) are looking for wisdom, grace and direction. As we age, we have an opportunity to pave the way for the younger generations, to inspire, to give them a new way of living that transcends outdated stereotypes.

As we age, remember that it isn't a time to lament the loss of youth, but rather a time for greater opportunities, greater health, connection, and especially inspiration. I believe we need to recognise our aging years as a privilege: if for no other reason, consider those in our community who have died prematurely through illness or accident. They did not have the opportunity or privilege of developing the wrinkles and stripes of years of living that they may have wished for themselves. Practising 'grateful aging' might be another way of considering it: the scientific reasoning behind this concept is that we can live longer when we appreciate the aging process (Schlitz, 2017). So, when your birthday comes around, enjoy the time it might take you to blow out all your candles. Embrace and capitalise on this phase of your life, because the benefits are enormous and powerful – for your health and wellbeing, and for those of others.

91. Don't act your age – act younger

Now, while I've just been telling you about the importance of embracing your age, there's also great merit in acting a little juvenile from time to time. Katharine Weber of Winnipeg, Canada, has some wonderful wisdom to teach us about the secret to a long, healthy and full life. She lived to the ripe young age of 108 with almost no health complaints, passing away in 2017. Her number-one secret was never to act her age. Her family attests to this. Her son, Thomas, said that at age 102, Katharine danced at her granddaughter's wedding and often flew to Ottawa and Vancouver to visit family up to that age. Born in 1909, Katharine was a child when the tanks first rolled across French battlefields in WWI. She lived through general strikes, pandemics, two world wars, and cold wars (Glassman, 2014), yet she retained a young and whimsical world view.

Having a young mindset is also evident in the Okinawan people of Japan. I've mentioned these marvellous people elsewhere in this book with regard to their diet. The region of Okinawa has the longest-living people in the world. Their philosophy is that residents are considered to be children until they reach the age of 55. Then, when they reach their ninety-seventh birthday, a ritual called *kajimaya* proclaims a return to their youth. Similarly, in Sardinia, Italy, there's an entrenched culture of youth and capability: age is celebrated, and people often work into their 90s. The traditional *kent'annos* greeting ('may you live to be 100') is common among the residents.

When you're next skipping down the shopping aisles, don't be deterred if someone tells you to act your age – just keep skipping!

92. Travel and explore new territory

Yes! Finally, a big-ticket item for your health and longevity. The key to this healthy strategy is simply experiencing new horizons, wherever they may be, while taking a break from your routine – even exploring your own back yard with a fresh perspective. However, let's talk about the broader concept of travel where you pack your bags, travel a reasonable distance from home and disconnect from your usual life. Australians are fans of travel, especially overseas travel, so we have an understanding of the therapeutic benefits. The ABS revealed that in 2012, 8.2 million residents (about a third of the country's population) left Australian shores for places like New Zealand, Thailand, United States, United Kingdom, Singapore, and Malaysia (Australia Post, 2016).

Let's look at the physical, mental and emotional benefits derived from travelling. A study commissioned by the Global Commission on Aging and Transamerica Center for Retirement Studies, in conjunction with the US Travel Association, found that adults who took a holiday twice a year were less likely to experience heart disease or heart attacks and had a 20% lower risk of death (Erskine, 2013). Then there's the argument that travel markedly reduces stress levels. Now, don't laugh in disbelief if you're a traveller who has ever lost your baggage, missed a connecting flight or forgotten your passport and experienced a meltdown as a result. These distresses are outweighed by the benefits. One study reveals that time away from work on a vacation reduces physical complaints and enhances sleep quality and mood, compared to pre-travel conditions. Admittedly, these are described as short-term benefits. But, hey, perhaps that shortcoming is another good reason to travel regularly (Chen & Petrick, 2013). Your brain also improves with the experience of travel. When you're adapting to new situations, meeting new people and developing global and cultural awareness, you're sharpening the grey matter. Travel is known to nurture a sense of greater openness and emotional stability (Zimmerman & Neyer, 2013).

But you don't need to have the travel mania of a Marco Polo or Captain Cook. A few days away at a beach or rainforest retreat within a few hours' drive of home has the same benefits as mentioned above. Then there's your own back yard. Refer to the earlier heading *A daily five-minute dose of journalling* for Julia Cameron's (2002) recommendations about tapping into your creative self through 'artist's dates'. Seeing the familiar through fresh eyes can be fun and provide a new perspective. As a medicine for longevity, travel, both near and far, is worth experiencing.

93. An attitude of gratitude

I'd like to share with you the significance and power behind the quality of being grateful. We all show gratitude in our own ways and what follows will, I hope, help you appreciate and want to express more deeply and often this attitude of gratitude.

When I read Dr John Demartini's book, *The Gratitude Effect* (2008), I was brought to tears – not of distress, but of joy in coming to a realisation at just how simple yet powerful genuine gratitude can be in supporting our emotional wellbeing and our relationships, and with manifesting what we would like to achieve in this life. True gratitude is an absolute appreciation for life. Demartini suggests we start each day by counting our blessings. He tells us that as we get out of bed in the morning, to think about what and who we can be authentically grateful for on this day. This attitude of gratitude is not a 'positive-thinking whitewash'. Far from it. It's a way of experiencing new levels of creativity and inspiration that will awaken our hidden potential. Demartini believes that when we are truly grateful for what we have, the Universe in its abundant generosity will give us more. Gratitude begets gratitude. When we are grateful for life, we open the gateway of our heart. While the morning offers us this opportunity to express thanks for what is to come, another opportunity is offered at the close of each day just before going to sleep: being thankful for whatever the day has presented to us. I like to take this evening time to do a review of my day and look back on all the events (both significant and small) and see how I can be grateful for that event or that person in my life. It may be that I'm reviewing the moment a car cut me off in the merging lane, or the perceived indifference of someone close to me to something that was important to me. In coming from a place of gratitude, the former event could well be a message about the need for patience and understanding, the latter a lesson in humility: thank you for both those learnings. The 'good' things too, need reviewing – a comfy bed, bountiful food, a family to love and be loved by, a smile from a stranger, being alive, being healthy. These are things not to be taken for granted, but rather, opportunities to exercise gratefulness.

And what I usually find happens is that I soon drift off to sleep in a state of gratitude, having a good night's sleep, waking refreshed and ready to start the next new day. Scientific research has found that expressing gratitude can have "dramatic and lasting effects in a person's life" by lowering blood pressure, improving the immune system, allowing for better sleep (as I've experienced) and enhancing levels of good cholesterol (Emmons, 2015).

If gratitude is a medicine for coping and thriving through the struggles in our lives, then the following is a powerful example. This remarkable woman who, despite or perhaps because of life's extreme challenges, knows the power of gratitude. As mentioned earlier in the book, ultra-marathoner Turia Pitt suffered burns to 64% of her body when she was caught in a bushfire in 2011. In her inspirational book *Unmasked* (2018), she says she starts each day with gratitude, explaining that when we're in that state, it's impossible to have any other negative sentiment. "You can't be grateful and angry at the same time, or grateful and bitter, or grateful and sad" (Pitt & Corbett, 2018: 265). These are wise words from a courageous and resilient young woman. While we can't control the actions and thoughts of others or necessarily escape seemingly random events in our lives, we do have control over our responses to these events, as Turia Pitt so wisely reveals. Gratitude, it would seem, is a powerful and rewarding place to start and finish each day.

94. Gratitude for your body

Now, you're probably wondering how this is different from the general attitude of gratitude discussed above. I came across a Facebook post (Brightside, 2016) that brought me to tears of gratitude for the amazing wisdom within our bodies that was expressed so well in this post. It outlined nine somewhat strange yet marvellous things that our bodies do automatically as a form of defence against potential harm. One related to yawning which is designed to cool down our brain and prevent overheating. Another wonderful automatic response – and one that really got gratitude going for my body responses – is what is called the myoclonic jerks.

You might know that response when you fall asleep very quickly and then jump awake. When you fall asleep rapidly, your breathing slows considerably, your pulse reduces slightly and your muscles become relaxed. In its infinite wisdom, the body perceives these signs as emulating impending death, so it jolts you awake to keep you alive! Another phenomenon is loss of memory which can sometimes occur following unpleasant experiences. It is the body's way of deleting those terrible moments as a sort of self-preservation measure. You may well have other examples of the body's innate ability to look after us. This marvellous inner wisdom, among other responses, was a real light-bulb moment of gratitude for me.

Alongside the beautiful wisdom within, my gratitude go-to person, Dr John Demartini (2018b), offers great insights into having gratitude for the physical aspects of our bodies. Many of us (myself included) dislike certain aspects of our bodies: perhaps our thighs are too large, our lips too thin, that front tooth sits funny, our feet are 'weird', and so on. Often, this perception is triggered by comparing ourselves to unrealistic images of the 'perfect body'. We all have things we like and dislike about our bodies, even supermodels! But as Demartini tells us, our physical bodies are "the greatest art form that exists on this planet", with the balance of likes and dislikes creating a perfect symmetry, or what Demartini describes as "a magnificently structured temple of sacred architecture" (2018b). The things we despise and the aspects we admire serve us because these likes and dislikes of our bodies create a unique balance to keep us growing (likes) and to keep us humble (dislikes). For instance, if we had only aspects that we admired about ourselves, we would develop an overly inflated ego and become proud, alienating ourselves from others.

So, how do we get to that state of gratitude for our physical bodies? The answer lies in asking ourselves how each aspect of our bodies serves us. Keep asking the question to the point of feeling absolute gratitude for every part of your body. In recognising the majesty and grandeur of our bodies, we begin to view them through a new lens of awe and gratitude.

Recognising and being grateful for the inner wisdom and outer magnificence of our bodies will add some healthy years to our lives.

95. Have faith

I'm not talking here about blind faith or even religious faith necessarily. For some, there is a belief in some form of higher power. My research has uncovered evidence to suggest that having faith in something beyond yourself is associated with longevity. 'Blue Zones®', a term trademarked by Dan Buettner, are geographic locations where the inhabitants have exceptionally long lifespans. It's been determined through Blue Zones studies that trust in a divine power and/or belonging to some form of faith-based community is a contributing factor to centenarians' physical health and longevity. Blue Zones research also reveals that attending faith-based services each week adds between four and 14 years of life expectancy (Blue Zones®, 2016). A University of Maryland Medical Center study suggests that those with strong religious or spiritual beliefs heal faster from surgery, experience less anxiety and depression, enjoy lower blood pressure, and cope better with chronic illnesses like arthritis, diabetes, heart disease, and cancer (Ewald, 2012). Katherine Weber, the centenarian who lived to 108, didn't focus on death but rather found peace in her belief in a higher power and the goodness of people (Glassman, 2014). In the publication *Leslie Beck's Longevity Diet* (Beck, 2010), researchers noted the importance of believing in something beyond ourselves.

Irrespective of a religious belief, it's tapping into the power of belief and faith that's the significant factor, whether it's getting involved in a community, volunteering for a cause or simply finding peace in nature (Ewald, 2012).

96. Lose track of time and be present

There's nothing more effective in stopping or slowing down the aging process than just being in the moment: being present, not thinking about the past or the future. Some might even call it daydreaming. Hungarian psychologist Mihaly Csikszentmihalyi uses the term 'flow' to describe this state – a highly focused mental state and immersion in activities such as work, play and art. Csikszentmihalyi argues that when you're in this state of flow, it opens up time. It's like a heightened state in which you experience greater inner clarity, have a greater arousal state, a knowingness to the task at hand, a timelessness in which hours will pass like minutes, and an intrinsic motivation irrespective of the task and its ease or difficulty. You've probably experienced this sense of flow yourself in the past. For example, you may recall a time when you were so immersed in what you were doing – whether a work-related task, playing a game or any activity – when you suddenly looked up and said, 'Oh wow, where has the time gone?' Csikszentmihalyi describes this flow as the secret to happiness. When you're on purpose or 'in flow', you cannot be apathetic. Apathy reflects a lack of interest or indifference. Flow or presence is apathy's opposite. While Csikszentmihalyi's model refers primarily to those who are seeking to undertake a big challenge or demanding skill, I believe that this state of flow or 'being present', as I have interpreted it, can be practised in any given moment if you put your mind to it. In a formal interpretation of flow, Csikszentmihalyi suggests that important factors to experience a sense of flow involve formulating clear objectives to what you want to achieve. This allows you to shift from what you can do, to what you are capable of or wish to achieve.

Another great contemporary mind on this issue is Dr John Demartini (The Values Factor, 2013). He states that the border between being supported and being challenged is where maximal emotional growth occurs. Demartini invites us to reflect on our day each evening and revisit all the events that made up our day. If we were challenged in any way, look for where we were equally supported. It's there he claims that we are all given an equal measure of support and challenge at any given time. It's just a matter of bringing it to our own attention. If we were supported in any way, look for the hidden challenges to create a perceptual balance. It is the intersection of these two powerful forces where human beings are at their most powerful: having an appreciation of both the 'good' and 'bad' in our lives helps us to be in a state of gratitude and presence. So, if you've got something specific you'd like or need to achieve, then being in a state of flow, as Csikszentmihalyi argues, is the way to go. But I believe it's also a tool that can be used at any time. Perhaps your objective is just to immerse yourself in being present and still. Set your objective and make sure you have a balance of challenging yourself sufficiently to extend yourself. For instance, you might decide that your objective is to be still and present for up to 15 minutes without your mind racing away from you into past regrets or future worries. Whatever you decide, it's best to choose a time frame and goal you haven't experienced previously or for some time. By applying Csikszentmihalyi's theory, the objective – 15 minutes of being still and present – is clear, and your balance of challenge and ability would seem to be 'doable' and realistic. When you're in flow, nothing matters, time stands still, and you find a moment of eternal youth and presence.

97. Meditate

I've referred to meditation previously in these pages, but let's take a closer look at the healthy benefits of meditating. Contrary to some folks' opinions, meditation is not a difficult art; it's not complex or necessarily time-consuming. Indeed, it's only as difficult or as easy as you choose it to be. According to Dr John Demartini (2014a), it's wise to master the use of your mind and develop a state of practical focus. Meditation can be done anywhere at any time (not while you're in charge of machinery though, be it plane, train, truck, car, ride-on mower, etc.). Your body position is not so important either but getting comfortable makes sense.

The following key points might make all the difference to a successful meditation experience. Firstly, if meditation is a new experience, use a comfortable chair to ease your way into the process. The second important element is a timer: iPhones and Android phones have built-in timers, or you can download the free app 'Insight Timer'. Thirdly, bring your attention to your breath, breathing naturally. And finally, when your mind wanders, which it inevitably will, gently bring your attention back to your breath (Bailey, 2013).

The important outcome in the meditative state is for your mind to become present, poised, purposeful, powerful, and patient. Demartini believes that there are two types of meditation: creature meditation and creative meditation. Creature meditation involves a passive receptivity to the Universe in which you experience gratitude for all that is and recognise the supreme order and balance of the Universe. This allows you to tune out the 'noise' (the fears, angers, resentments, busyness, and so on). This state of gratitude and presence calms the brain, allowing your breathing and your mind to be in balance, and allowing you to be fully present in the moment. In this state, you will be open to inspired messages. Demartini advocates that you write these messages down as they come to you, so have a pen and paper or your notes section of your iPhone handy so you don't miss the gems as they emerge in the passive creature state of meditation.

Creative meditation focuses on the finer details of the messages and information you receive in the passive creature state. In this creative state you shift into becoming an active participant in the meditation process, concentrating on what inspires you so that you can bring it into your reality. As you focus on what inspires you, you bring ever-greater detail to your mind. This then forms the basis of your goals and aspirations. The benefits to your life and health are enormous. As Demartini asserts, by mastering your mind in this way, you reduce your stress levels, which in turn allows you to pursue what you are truly meant to do in this life.

Additionally, according to US research from the University of Waterloo, just 10 minutes of mindful meditation can reduce anxiety while improving focus (Grant, 2017). Blood pressure and cortisol levels (stress hormone) were said to have significantly reduced in participants who practised Buddhist meditation daily over a four-month trial (Corbett, 2014). A key aspect of Buddhist meditation is that it encompasses practices to develop mindfulness (*sati*) and concentration (*samadhi*). Buddhists believe that everything comes from the mind, suggesting that our physical, emotional, mental, and spiritual health are directly linked to our minds. Buddhists practise the art of detaching themselves from their thoughts, creating a state of stillness which ultimately leads to an understanding of self and to enlightenment (Graham, 2007).

If you have ever tried meditation and noticed how your mind seemed to run a constant fast-paced cinematic experience with no gaps or silences, then you're not alone. My understanding is that it is the art of simply having an experience and doing your best to be still while acknowledging the passing parade of thoughts. Persistence and consistency are important here. So, take a few moments for yourself each day to be totally present and grateful. Witness your genius emerge, and as Demartini says, record it, act on it and know that you've not only reduced any tension in mind and body, but opened up a gateway to a purpose-filled life (Demartini, 2014a).

98. Tai chi

The first time I witnessed tai chi in action was in a park. A small group of people dressed in black were all moving their upper bodies in slow but deliberate motions and in perfect unison. It was captivating but somewhat bewildering. I knew it as tai chi, but I had no understanding or appreciation then for the skill and control involved, let alone its meditative qualities or its powerful implications for health and longevity. The full term and spelling is *taijiquan* (pronounced 'tie jee chwenn') and it is derived from Taoist philosophy. Taoism is an ancient Chinese nature-based ideology. As the Taoists explain, before the Universe existed there was a state of *wu chi* (no polarity), a void or nothingness, inferring that there was no differentiation. With a change in state came tai chi, which literally translates as 'great polarity' – the opposite poles, or yin and yang, which gave rise to all things and processes. The 'quan' (chwenn) element of the practice literally means 'fist' and is the martial arts component of this ancient practice. But it's not simply about fighting. The philosophy was inspired by the bird species, the crane, but also close observation of all animal and plant life. Taoists observed plants growing and animals fighting and studied their nature, how they moved, how they thought, how they survived – their physical, mental and spiritual yin and yang – and adapted these observations for themselves. This ancient cultural treasure has been shared with the Western world to help us understand and benefit from the balance of yin and yang to enrich our lives by manifesting change in ourselves (Internal Gardens Tai Chi, 2012).

The theory behind tai chi is that by integrating the mind, body and spirit we can overcome the limitations of our bodies by incorporating intention to guide our movements. These gentle movements are said to reduce stress and promote serenity, while supporting a range of health conditions such as backaches, neck complaints, high blood pressure, tumours, and breathing problems (Wagland, nd). Those who practise the art of tai chi are said to develop greater balance, have reduced pain, experience increased immunity, enjoy an elevated aerobic capacity, and benefit from an overall enhanced quality of life. Tai chi is especially wonderful for relieving or eliminating stress. As with deep breathing discussed elsewhere, it works closely with the autonomic nervous system to return you to a calm and balanced state (David Cui, personal communication, 29 July 2018).

Most significantly, especially in the context of this book, scientific research into this ancient Chinese art form suggests that it may also slow the aging process by boosting a certain type of stem cell. Three groups of young people were tested in a year-long retrospective study, with the participants engaged in tai chi, brisk walking or no exercise, the results then compared for their rejuvenating and anti-aging effects. Known as a CD34+ protein, this stem cell is involved in cell self-renewal. The results of the study revealed that the group involved in the tai chi had a significantly higher number of the CD34+ cells. The researchers argue that tai chi prompts dilation of blood vessels and thus increased blood flow. The studied group was aged under 25 years, chosen because of their better cell-renewing ability when compared with the older population, and because of the reduced risk of participants having chronic illnesses or medications that might interfere with the test results. While the researchers contend that further study is required on diverse and older populations, the results are encouraging that this is a worthwhile anti-aging exercise, especially if they can be reproduced in the less-young among us (American Association for the Advancement of Science, 2014).

Perhaps we need look no further than Chinese-born Lu Zijian, a famous martial artist and master of the Taoist tai chi philosophy. He died just one month before his hundred and nineteenth birthday in 2012, having remained active and agile until then (Zijian, 2016).

99. Find moments of awe

As I began writing and researching for this topic, the world was focusing its attention on 12 young Thai soccer players and their coach trapped one kilometre underground and four kilometres from the entrance in a narrow and darkened cave in Tham Luang, Thailand (Hodge, 2018). The incident had all the hallmarks of a perilous rescue mission. When initially found by two British cave divers nine days after going missing, on 23 June 2018, the boys and their coach were huddled on a ledge, calm but in a weakened state after days in isolation, with diminishing oxygen, darkness and little or no food. The early monsoon rains were flooding the cave system and causing strong currents, hampering any rescue attempt. Time was against the rescuers and the 13 trapped souls. None could swim, and they had no diving experience. Yet, despite the odds against them, the boys and their coach were eventually rescued successfully, but for one tragedy, a Thai navy SEAL who died from a lack of oxygen while delivering supplies to the missing group.

This momentous event moved me and many people around the world as we followed the media's reporting of the drama. It was an awe-inspiring event on several levels: firstly, the fact that two British cave divers managed to find the boys and coach alive and in good spirits after so many days trapped; secondly, that support, equipment and supplies were swift and broad across the global community with diving experts, local and international military support, medical experts, local and overseas volunteers all providing support in their own unique ways, while the rest of us prayed and provided spiritual backing; thirdly, while essentially a military operation it was led chiefly by civilian authorities and foreign experts, a uniquely decentralised operation in a country that is ruled by a military junta; and finally, the rescued themselves surviving relatively unscathed physically and, we hope, emotionally. Each of these elements in isolation demonstrates the spirit of humanity and collectively, they arouse a sense of awe at the sheer *attempt*, let alone the accomplishment!

Awe can be defined as that feeling we get in the presence of something larger than ourselves that challenges our usual way of seeing the world and engenders in us a sense of smallness, not in a shameful or self-doubting way but rather in an interconnected way with others (Breines, 2016). Moreover, a study called *Awe, the Small Self, and Prosocial Behaviour* revealed that a sense of wonder and awe promotes a sense of altruism, loving-kindness and magnanimity among us (Piff *et al*, 2015). The Thai cave mission certainly seems to have galvanised many millions around the world as we witnessed something much greater than ourselves, and humanity at its absolute best. We hope, of course, that our sense of wonder and awe would not have to be kindled too often by such events.

Sources of awe are frequently found in what we might perceive as the commonplace and everyday events in our lives. Mother Nature supplies us with opportunities to experience these peak moments – sunrise and sunset, a rippling creek, majestic mountains, trees, the intricacies of flowers... Then there's those around us: a daughter's laughter, our ability to breathe deeply, a baby born, the close of a life well lived. Music, art and religion are also fuel for awe if we take the time to recognise these peak moments, even if they are only fleeting. We may, however, need to have our antennae up so we don't miss them, but once we ignite our awareness to the wonder around us, we may be pleasantly surprised to discover just how many opportunities there are to be wonderstruck (Bergland, 2015).

Alongside the altruism and sense of connection that we derive from awe, there are several physical health benefits to be gained from this positive emotion. Research undertaken in 2015 by the University of California has shown that when we experience awe, it positively affects our health with a reduction in inflammation and the lowering of the risk of heart disease, type 2 diabetes and Alzheimer's. Researcher Jennifer Stellar and her colleagues at the University of Toronto conducted two studies, the first on the connection between health and positive emotions. They tested saliva samples from their subjects for the molecule interlukin-6 (IL-6) that promotes inflammation in the body. The results revealed that positive emotional experiences produced lower levels of IL-6. The second study centred on the subjects exposed to a range of positive emotions – joy, contentment, pride, and awe – followed by more saliva tests for the IL-6 molecule. Experiencing a sense of awe had the greatest influence in reducing this disease-inducing molecule, the researchers suggesting that experiencing awe has a direct influence on health and life expectancy (Makin, 2015).

If you'd like to experience more awe for a longer life, then the Greater Good Science Center has compiled four practices to enhance these experiences. The first strategy they call 'Awe Narrative' which invites us to write down our awe experiences, the exercise said to lift the doldrums, enhance the experience further and foster our desire for altruism. Next, they invite us to take an 'Awe Walk' even in places we may be very familiar with, experiencing these spaces as if seeing them for the first time. Being in the right frame of mind (being present, iPhone switched off, drawing on all our senses and breathing deeply) will invoke a sense of wonder and inspiration. Thirdly, watching an 'awe video' such as a panoramic view to gain a perspective on our relatively small place in the Universe can be visually enthralling, or watching an act of exceptional heroism that could expand our understanding of human potential, will tap into the awe within. Finally, reading an 'awe story' has the capacity to alter the way we see the world, perhaps allowing us to put any mundane concerns to one side and appreciate others' challenges and triumphs (Breines, 2016). Irish singer/songwriter Van Morrison released an inspiring song back in 1985 called *Sense of Wonder*. It was the culmination of a period of spiritual awakening for the artist – rebirth, meditation, ecstasy, humility, and bliss – his lyrics invoking a sense of wonder for his Celtic roots (Puterbaugh, 1985). Perhaps we can take a leaf from Morrison's song sheets and find moments of awe and wonder in our own circumstances, knowing that altruism and a healthier life are wonderful by-products.

100. Simple homespun wisdom from supercentenarians

I'd like to close these 100 topics by giving the last word to some of our supercentenarians: the wonderful folk who've made it to that magic 100 years and beyond. They are, of course, the inspiration and driving force for this book.

> "Always eat when you're hungry, always drink when you're dry, always sleep when you are sleepy, don't stop breathing or you'll die"—Dexter Kruger, aged 108 years, 1910– (Edmistone, 2017).
>
> "Good clean living, no smoking, no drinking, but lots of cups of tea"—Phyllis Lee, aged 110 years, 1907–2017 (Edmistone, 2017).
>
> "I might be 100 but I don't feel 100. I don't stop to think of my age at all, I just live my life how it comes. You wake up, you get out of bed and you get on with your work! If you live a life, live a happy one and don't look for trouble"—Winifred Warden, aged 101 years, 1917– (Edmistone, 2017).
>
> "My age has no impact. I'm still working like I did before. I always went swimming at noon, and I still exercise today. The diet is very important. How you live is very important. All of those are very important to what causes disease"—Dr Fred Kummerow, aged 101 years when quoted, 1914–2017 (Peat, 2015).
>
> "We all remember how as children, when we were having fun, we often forgot to eat or sleep. I believe that we

can keep that attitude as adults, too. It's best not to tire the body with too many rules such as lunchtime and bedtime"—Dr Shigeaki Hinohara, aged 105 years when quoted, 1911–2017 (Gillett, 2017).

"I think you should push back from the table when you're still hungry"—Walter Breuning, aged 114 years, 1896–2011 (Wedeman, 2016).

"I try not to worry, I just try to live...And I try to have enough trust and confidence in myself to deal with things as they come"—Katharine Weber, aged 102 years when quoted, 1909–2017 (Glassman, 2014).

"You should stop just when you know you can eat a little more"—Fauja Singh, aged 105 years when quoted, 1911– (Menon, 2016).

"I don't fight it, I live it"—Flossie Dickey, aged 110 years, 1906–2016 (Shah, 2016).

Acknowledgements

To my dear family and friends for supporting me with your interest, ideas and simply lending an ear to 'another great chapter idea' as it came to me.

To Rae Bryce, friend, neighbour and retired teacher who undertook the initial read and edit of my manuscript, providing honest and welcome feedback and commentary.

To my editor, Gail Tagarro, for your patience, brilliant insights and editing expertise. You've polished my dream.

To cartoonist, Sean Leahy, for drawing out the humour so acutely and bringing the topics to life.

To the giants whose shoulders I have stood on. Your wisdom and guiding principles have been the inspiration for this book. Among them: Hippocrates, David Gillespie, Dr John Demartini, Dr Robert Lustig, Dr Libby Weaver, and Professor Brene Brown.

To the healthy supercentenarians whose marvellous and inspiring stories have proven that anything is possible.

Reference List

ABC Radio, (2013, 30 July). Bruce Lourie and Rick Smith studied the toxins of everyday life [Radio Program]. *Conversations with Richard Fidler*. Retrieved from http://www.abc. net.au/local/stories/2013/07/30/3814042.htm

Abdel-Aal, E.M., Akhtar, H., Zaheer, K. & Ali, R. (2013, April). Dietary Sources of Lutein and Zeaxanthin Carotenoids and Their Role in Eye Health. *Nutrients, 5:4*. Retrieved from https://www.ncbi.nlm.nih.gov/pmc/articles/PMC3705341/

American Association for the Advancement of Science, The (2014, 28 May). Can Tai Chi Slow the Ageing Process? *Eureka Alert*. Retrieved from https://www.eurekalert. org/pub_releases/2014-05/ctco-ctc052814.php

Andre, D. (2016). In fibromyalgia patients, music therapy can reduce pain, depression, anxiety, and improve sleep. *Bell Marra Health*. Retrieved from http://www.belmarrahealth. com/in-fibromyalgia-patients-music-therapy-can-reduce-pain-depression-anxiety-and-improve-sleep/

Anthony, N. (2017). 5 celebrities that endorse bone broth. *Nothing But Broth*. Retrieved from https:// nothingbutbroth.com/celebrities-endorse-bone-broth/

Aroniadis O. & Brandt L. (2013). Fecal Microbiota Transplantation Past, Present and Future, Current Opinion in Gastroenterology. In *Melbourne Faecal Microbial Transplant*, 29(1):79-84. Retrieved from http://www.melbournefmt.com.au/

Asher, N., (2017, 9 May). Faecal transplants could cause recipients to take on donors' traits: expert, *ABC News*, Retrieved http://www.abc.net.au/news/2017-05-09/faecal-transplant-side-effects-explored-at-conference/8510270

Australia Post. (2016, 22 August). Travel Trends – How Australians Travel, *AustPost Travel Team*. Retrieved from https://auspost.com.au/travel-essentials/how-australians-travel

Australian Eggs Limited. (2018a). *Healthy Ageing*. Retrieved from https://www.australianeggs.org.au/nutrition/healthy-ageing/

Australian Eggs Limited. (2018b). *Egg Myths.* Retrieved from https://www.australianeggs.org.au/nutrition/egg-myths/

Australian Government Department of Health. (2018, 24 April). *Health Warnings: Tobacco*. Retrieved from http://www.health.gov.au/internet/main/publishing.nsf/content/tobacco-warn

Australian Medical Association. (2018, 7 January). *Nutrition – 2018*. Retrieved from https://ama.com.au/position-statement/nutrition-2018

Australian Securities & Investments Commission (ASIC). (2018, 22 March). *Money Smart: Credit Card Debt Clock.* Retrieved from https://www.moneysmart.gov.au/borrowing-and-credit/credit-cards/credit-card-debt-clock

Australian Thyroid Foundation Ltd. (2018). *Iodine Deficiency & Nutrition.* Retrieved from https://thyroidfoundation.org.au/Iodine-Deficiency

Axe, J. (2018). *Bone Broth Benefits for Digestion, Arthritis and Cellulite.* Retrieved from https://draxe.com/the-healing-power-of-bone-broth-for-digestion-arthritis-and-cellulite/

Axe, J. (2018a). *Pink Himalayan Salt Benefits that Make It Superior to Table Salt.* Retrieved from https://draxe.com/pink-himalayan-salt/

Axelsson, A., Tubbs, E., Mecham, B., Chacko, S., Nenonen, H.A., Tang, Y., Fahey, J.W., Derry, J.M.J., Wollheim, C.B., Wierup, N., Haymond, M.W., Friend, S.H., Mulder, H., and Rosengren, A.H. (2017, 14 June). Sulforaphane reduces hepatic glucose production and improves glucose control in patients with type 2 diabetes. *Science Translational Medicine*, 9(394). Retrieved from http://stm.sciencemag.org/content/9/394/eaah4477

Bailey, C. (2013, 17 May). Meditation/Mindfulness Guide: Everything you need to start meditating. *A Life of Productivity*. Retrieved from https://alifeofproductivity.com/meditation-guide/

Baraz, J. & Alexander, S. (2010, 1 February). The Helper's High. *Greater Good Magazine*. Retrieved from https://greatergood.berkeley.edu/article/item/the_helpers_high

Barth, B. (2014, 5 June). Did the Tiananmen Square protests lead to more democracy in China? *Wilfried Martens Centre for European Studies*. Retrieved from https://www.martenscentre.eu/blog/did-tiananmen-square-protests-lead-more-democracy-china

Basis, H. (2018, 14 March). Orthopaedic Reflexology, *LinkedIn*, 14 March. Retrieved from https://www.linkedin.com/pulse/orthopedic-reflexology-hagar-basis

Bauer, B.A. (2015, 23 September). What is Reflexology? Can It Relieve Stress? *Mayo Clinic*. Retrieved from https://www.mayoclinic.org/healthy-lifestyle/consumer-health/expert-answers/what-is-reflexology/faq-20058139

Baxter, R.A. (2014, 26 August). Dancing With The Scars: A Plastic Surgeon's Tango Fandango. *The Art Behind Plastic Surgery*. Retrieved from http://www.drbaxter.com/blog/blog/post/dancing-with-the-scars-a-plastic-surgeons-tango-fandango

Beck, L. (2010). Leslie Beck's Longevity Diet: The Power Of Food To Slow Aging And Maintain Optimal Health And Energy, Penguin: Canada.

Bee, P. (2018, 4 June). Happy Feet. *The Australian*, Life, p. 10.

Bell, L. (2017, 14 August). Escape Tech: What Is A Digital Detox, How And Why To Do One And Where To Do It, *Forbes Tech #LifeHacks*. Retrieved from https://www.forbes.com/sites/leebelltech/2017/08/14/escape-tech-what-is-a-digital-detox-how-and-why-to-do-one-and-where-to-do-it/2/#416a6db87723

Bergland, C. (2015, 20 May). The Power of Awe: A Sense of Wonder Promotes Loving-Kindness. *Psychology Today*. Retrieved from https://www.psychologytoday.com/au/blog/the-athletes-way/201505/the-power-awe-sense-wonder-promotes-loving-kindness

Beuttner, D. (2016, 10 November), Power 9®: Reverse Engineering Longevity. *Blue Zones*. Retrieved from https://www.bluezones.com/2016/11/power-9/

Binding, L. (2016, 20 April). Sweet Potatoes Will 'Help You To Live To 100', BBC1 Documentary Discovers. *International Business Times*. Retrieved from http://www.ibtimes.co.uk/sweet-potatoes-will-help-you-live-100-bbc1-documentary-discovers-1555887

Bolen, J.S. (2014). Goddesses in Older Women: Archetypes in Women Over Fifty: Becoming a Juicy Crone. Harper Paperbacks.

Booth, M. (2013, 20 June). The Okinawa diet – could it help to live to 100? *The Guardian*. Retrieved from https://www.theguardian.com/lifeandstyle/2013/jun/19/Japanese-diet-to-live-to-100

Breast Cancer Network Australia. (2018). *Breast Awareness.* Retrieved from https://www.bcna.org.au/breast-health-awareness/breast-awareness/

Breines, J. (2016, 8 March). Four Awe-Inspiring Activities. *Greater Good Magazine.* Retrieved from https://greatergood.berkeley.edu/article/item/four_awe_inspiring_activities

Brightside. (2016). *9 Strange Things Your Body Does That You Never Knew Were Defense Mechanisms.* Retrieved from https://brightside.me/wonder-curiosities/9-strange-things-your-body-does-that-you-never-knew-were-defense-mechanisms-263110/

Britton, K. (2017). How to start journaling and practice self-care, daily! *I Heart Wellness.* Retrieved from http://www.iheartwellness.com/how-to-start-to-journal-daily/

Brown, B. (2015). Daring Greatly : How the Courage to be Vulnerable Transforms the Way We Live, Love, Parent, and Lead, New York, USA: Penguin Putnam Inc.

Buettner, D. (2016, 10 November). Power 9®: Reverse Engineering Longevity. *Blue Zones.* Retrieved from https://bluezones.com/2016/11/power-9/

Butler, K. (2015, 9 November). Enough Already With the Bone Broth Hype. *Mother Jones.* Retrieved from https://www.motherjones.com/environment/2015/11/truth-about-bone-broth/

Cameron, J. (2002). *The Artist's Way*, New York: Jeremy P. Tarcher/Putnam.

Cancer Council Australia. (2017, 11 December). *Breast Cancer.* Retrieved from https://www.cancer.org.au/about-cancer/early-detection/early-detection-factsheets/breast-cancer.html

Cancer Council Australia. (2018, 1 January). Breast Cancer Statistics, *Breast Cancer*. Retrieved from https://breast-cancer.canceraustralia.gov.au/statistics

Cancer Council Australia. (2018, 3 January). *Skin Cancer*. Retrieved from http://www.cancer.org.au/about-cancer/types-of-cancer/skin-cancer.html

Cancer Council Australia. (2016, January). National Cancer Control Policy. *Position Statement – Sun exposure and vitamin D – risk and benefits*. Retrieved from https://wiki.cancer.org.au/policy/Position_statement_-_Risks_and_benefits_of_sun_exposure#Sun_exposure_and_the_UV_Index

Cancer Council Australia. (2018, 30 January). *Bowel Cancer Statistics*. Retrieved from https://bowel-cancer.canceraustralia.gov.au/statistics

Carlson, R. (1997). Don't Sweat the Small Stuff... and it's all small stuff. Milsons Point, Australia: Bantam.

Carrano, J. (2017, 23 November). Australia's waistline fifth-largest in OECD as obesity and overweight rates soar. *Brisbane Times: Healthcare*. Retrieved from https://www.brisbanetimes.com.au/healthcare/australias-waistline-fifthlargest-in-oecd-as-obesity-and-overweight-rates-soar-20171123-gzrfks.html

Cell Wellbeing. (2017). *Useful background information on the ever increasing dangers of EMF's and ELF's*. Retrieved from http://cell-wellbeing.com/useful-background-information-on-the-ever-increasing-dangers-of-emfs-and-elfs/

Center for Mindful Eating, The. (nd). *The Principles of Mindful Eating*. Retrieved from http://www.thecenterformindfuleating.org/Principles-Mindful-Eating

Charnetski, C.J., Brennan F.X. Jr. & Harrison, J.F. (1998). Effect of music and auditory stimuli on secretory immunoglobulin A (IgA). *Wilkes University, Pennsylvania. Retrieved from* https://www.ncbi.nlm.nih.gov/pubmed/10052073

Chen, C. & Petrick, J.F. (2013, 17 July). Health and Wellness Benefits of Travel Experiences. *Journal of Travel Research.* Retrieved from http://journals.sagepub. com/doi/abs/10.1177/0047287513496477

Cherkin, D., Sherman, K.J., Kahn, J., Wellman, R., Cook, A.J., Johnson, E., Erro. J., Delaney, K. & R.A. Deyo. (2011, 5 July). A Comparison of the Effects of 2 Types of Massage and Usual Care on Chronic Low Back Pain: A Randomized, Controlled Trial. *Annals of Internal Medicine*, 155(1): 1-9. Retrieved from http://annals.org/aim/search-results?q=massage%20therapy% 20back%20pain&allJournals=1&fl_IsJCA=false&SearchS ourceType=1&exPrm_qqq={!payloadDisMaxQParser%20 pf=Tags%20qf=Tags^0.0000001%20payloadFields=Tags%20 bf=}%22massage%20therapy%20back%20pain%22

Chung, H., Pamp, S.J., Hill, J.A., Surana, N.K., Edelman, S.M., Troy, E.B., Reading, N.C., Villablanca, E.J., Wang, S., Mora, J.R., Umesaki, Y., Mathis, D., Benoist, C., Relman, D.A. & Kasper, D.L. (2012, 22 June). Gut Immune Maturation Depends on Colonization with a Host-Specific Microbiota. *National Center for Biotechnology Information, Cell,* 149:7, pp. 1578-1593. Retrieved from https://www. ncbi.nlm.nih.gov/pmc/articles/PMC3442780/

Cityline. (2017, 14 June). 56 different names for sugars hiding on food labels. Cityline. Retrieved from https://www. cityline.tv/2017/06/14/56-names-sugars-havent-heard/

Clark, B., Kelly, J., Leggatt, J. & Mayoh, L. (2015, 1 August). 100 ways to live to 100: tips for a longer, healthier life. *The Mercury.* Retrieved from https://www.themercury.com.

au/lifestyle/ways-to-live-to-100-tips-for-a-longer-healthier-life/news-story/cc35f1f59f89b2d7104dd2bb6bd1caef

Cockburn, H. (2016, 7 September). Scientists find 'Key To Longevity' in Italian Village Where One In 10 People Live Beyond 100 Years. *Independent*. Retrieved from https://www.independent.co.uk/life-style/health-and-families/health-news/scientists-key-to-longevity-italy-acciaroli-centenarian-mediterranean-diet-a7230956.html

Cohen, R., Bavishi, C. & Rozanski, A. (2016, February/March). Purpose in Life and Its Relationship to All-Cause Mortality and Cardiovascular Events: A Meta-Analysis. *Psychosomatic Medicine*, 78:2, 122-133. Retrieved from https://journals.lww.com/psychosomaticmedicine/Citation/2016/02000/Purpose_in_Life_and_Its_Relationship_to_All_Cause.2.aspx

Cole, W. (2017, 6 December). Which Is Better For Your Gut — Apple Cider Vinegar Or Lemon Water? *MindBodyGreen*. Retrieved from https://www.mindbodygreen.com/articles/apple-cider-vinegar-vs-lemon-water-for-gut-health

Continence Foundation of Australia. (2018). *Bristol Stool Chart*. Retrieved from https://www.continence.org.au/pages/bristol-stool-chart.html

Conversation, The. (2018). Gut feeling: how your microbiota affects your mood, sleep and stress levels. *The Conversation*. Retrieved from http://theconversation.com/gut-feeling-how-your-microbiota-affects-your-mood-sleep-and-stress-levels-65107

Coppafeel. (2018). *Boob Check 101,* https://coppafeel.org/your-boobs/boob-check-101/

Corbett, H. (2014, 25 September). 25 Things That Will Keep You Young, *Redbook*. Retrieved from https://www.redbookmag.com/beauty/anti-aging/advice/g602/fight-aging/?slide=14

Corca, D. (2017). Daily Napping Could Help Save Your Life, *HuffPost*, https://www.huffingtonpost.com/damiana-corca/daily-napping-could-save-_b_9888338.html

Corliss, J. (2013, 20 November). *Eating nuts linked to healthier, longer life.* https://www.health.harvard.edu/blog/eating-nuts-linked-to-healthier-longer-life-201311206893

Corrado, M. (2015, 27 August). The Dark Side of Bone Broth. *Selene River Press.* Retrieved from https://www.seleneriverpress.com/the-dark-side-of-bone-broth/

Corriher, S.C. (nd). The Dangers of Non-Stick Cookware. *The Health Wyze Report.* Retrieved from https://healthwyze.org/reports/96-the-dangers-of-non-stick-cookware

Cosman, J. (2017, 27 February). The Amazing Benefits of Stretching. *Whole Body Health Physical Therapy.* Retrieved from http://www.wholebodyhealth-pt.com/wbhptblog/2017/2/20/the-amazing-benefits-of-stretching

Craik, F.I.M., Bialystok, E. & Freedman, M. (2010, 9 November). Neurology, Delaying the onset of Alzheimer disease Bilingualism as a form of cognitive reserve. *Neurology.* Retrieved from http://www.neurology.org/content/75/19/1726.short

Csikszentmihalyi, M. (2004). Flow, the secret to happiness. *TED2004.* Retrieved from https://www.ted.com/talks/mihaly_csikszentmihalyi_on_flow

CureJoy Editorial. (2016, 21 June). *The Correct Way Of Drinking Water As Per Ayurveda.* Retrieved from http://www.curejoy.com/content/the-right-way-of-drinking-water-as-per-ayurveda/

Dashiell, C. (2017, 14 April). Periodic check-ups key to baby boomer health and longevity. *David Geffen School of*

Medicine: Health News. Retrieved from http://medschool. ucla.edu/body.cfm?id=1158&action=detail&ref=1008

Datz, T. (2016). More exposure to vegetation linked with lower mortality rates in women. *Harvard T H Chan School of Public Health: News.* Retrieved from https://www.hsph.harvard. edu/news/press-releases/plants-death-rates-women/

de Hennezel, M. (2017). *Sex After Sixty: A French Guide to Loving Intimacy.* Brunswick, Victoria: Scribe Publications.

Deakin University. (2012, 16 November). *Vitamin D deficiency strikes one-third of Australians.* Retrieved from http:// www.deakin.edu.au/research/research-news/articles/ vitamin-d-deficiency-strikes-one-third-of-australians

Demartini, J.F. (1989). Demartini Value Determination & Application Processes™. *Demartini Institute.* Retrieved from www.DrDemartini.com

Demartini, J.F. (2008). *The Gratitude Effect*, Frenchs Forest, Australia: New Holland Publishers.

Demartini, J.F. (2009). The Breakthrough Experience: A Revolutionary New Approach to Personal Transformation. Carlsbad, United States: Hay House Inc.

Demartini, J.F. (2013). The Values Factor: The Secret to Creating an Inspired and Fulfilling Life, United States: Penguin Group.

Demartini, J.F. (2014, April). The Law of Meditation. *Demartini Institute.* Newsletters. Retrieved from https:// drdemartini.wistia.com/medias/mdc1o07c3p

Demartini, J.F. (2014a). The Art of Meditation. [Video clip]. *The Demartini Institute.* Retrieved from https:// drdemartini.wistia.com/medias/mdc1o07c3p

Demartini, J.F. (2015, 19 June). How To Get Out Of A Rut. *Demartini Institute Blog.* Retrieved from https://drdemartini.com/blog/get-out-of-a-rut/

Demartini, J.F. (2016, 22 April). Advice on Setting Goals With Values. *Demartini Institute Blog.* Retrieved from https://drdemartini.com/blog/setting-goals/

Demartini, J.F. (2017, 14 May). What to Look For When Seeking a Mentor or Coach.... *Demartini Institute Blog.* Retrieved from https://drdemartini.com/blog/seeking-mentor-coach/

Demartini, J.F. (2017a, 15 November). Free Your Finances to Avoid Debt. *Demartini Institute Blog.* Retrieved from https://drdemartini.com/blog/avoiding-debt/

Demartini, J.F. (2018, 28 June). *From Stress to Success.* [YouTube clip]. Retrieved from https://www.youtube.com/watch?time_continue=1&v=nwKCxS-9oX0

Demartini, J.F. (2018a). Demartini It! Solving Your Challenges. *Demartini Institute Blog.* Retrieved from https://drdemartini.com/demartini-it/dissolving-challenges/

Demartini, J.F. (2018b). Appreciating your physical body as it is.... *Demartini Institute Blog.* Retrieved from https://drdemartini.com/appreciating-physical-body/?utm_source=dlvr.it&utm_medium=facebook&utm_campaign=snug+corner

Demartini, J.F. (nd). The Benefits of Making Lists to Health. *Demartini Institute Blog.* https://drdemartini.com/writings_and_insights/the_benefits_of_making_lists_to_health

Department of Health. (2013, November). Reduce your risk: new national guidelines for alcohol consumption. Retrieved from http://www.alcohol.gov.au/internet/alcohol/publishing.nsf/Content/guide-adult

Department of Health & Human Services. (2013a, April). Milk. *Better Health Channel*. State Government of Victoria. Retrieved from https://www.betterhealth.vic.gov.au/health/healthyliving/milk

Department of Health & Human Services. (2013, January). Fish, *Better Health Channel*. State Government of Victoria. Retrieved from https://www.betterhealth. vic.gov.au/health/HealthyLiving/fish

Department of Health & Human Services. (2016, 21 June). The benefits of eating a variety of fruits and vegetables, *Better Health Channel*, State Government of Victoria. Retrieved from https://www. betterhealth.vic.gov.au/blog/blogcollectionpage/eat-a-rainbow

Department of Health & Human Services. (2017, April). Parkinson's disease. *Better Health Channel*, State Government of Victoria. Retrieved from https://www.betterhealth.vic.gov. au/health/conditionsandtreatments/parkinsons-disease

Dhami, P., Moreno, S. & DeSouza, J.F. (2015, 28 January). New Framework for Rehabilitation – fusion of cognitive and physical rehabilitation: the hope for dancing, *Frontiers in Psychology – Cognitive Science*. 5:1478. Retrieved from https://www.ncbi.nlm.nih.gov/pubmed/25674066

Di Donato, V. (2016, 30 November). Oldest living person credits longevity to raw eggs, independence. *CNN*. Retrieved from https://edition.cnn.com/2016/11/29/ health/oldest-living-person-emma-morano/index.html

Dolhun, R. (2018). What is Parkinson's? *Shake It Up Australia Foundation*. Retrieved from https:// shakeitup.org.au/understanding-parkinsons/

Donvito, T. (2018). 50 Easy Habits That Help You Live Longer, According to Science. *Reader's Digest*. Retrieved from https://www.rd.com/health/wellness/live-longer/

Drayer, L. (2017, 14 April). Are Eggs Healthy? *CNN.*
 Retrieved from https://edition.cnn.com/2017/04/14/
 health/eggs-healthy-food-drayer/index.html

Eadie, G.A. (1945). The Over-All Mental-Health Needs of
 the Industrial Plant, with Special Reference to War
 Veterans. *Mental Hygiene*, 29:1, 101-103. New York:
 National Committee for Mental Hygiene, Inc.

Edmistone, L. (2017, 9-10 December), Tales of the Century.
 The Courier-Mail, Q-Weekend, pp. 8-11.

Elias, N. (2013, 5 December). Ten Things Your Feet Say About Your
 Health, *Prevention*. Retrieved from https://www.prevention.com/
 life/g20499078/foot-pain-and-foot-fungus-feet-and-your-health/

Emmons, R.A. (2015, 25 November). Gratitude is Good
 Medicine. *UC Davis Medical Center*. Retrieved from
 http://www.ucdmc.ucdavis.edu/medicalcenter/
 features/2015-2016/11/20151125_gratitude.html

Erhmann, M. (1927). Desiderata. *Silkworth.net*. Retrieved
 from http://silkworth.net/pages/aa/desiderata.php

Erskine, C. (2013, 17 December). Travel is the Best
 Medicine, Study Finds. *Los Angeles Times.* Retrieved
 from http://articles.latimes.com/2013/dec/17/news/
 la-trb-travel-best-medicine-study-20131217

Ewald, J. (2012). The Important Relationship between Faith and
 Longevity. *Life + Health*. Retrieved from https://lifeandhealth.
 org/readandwatch/live/faith-and-longevity/14428.html

EyeMed. (2018). How a routine eye exam can save your life. *Eye Site
 on Wellness.* Retrieved from http://www.eyesiteonwellness.
 com/how-a-routine-eye-exam-can-save-your-life/

Fallon Morrell, S. (2014). *Nourishing Broth.* Grand Central Publishing.

Fitzgibbon, L. (2014, 31 August). Carb Confusion. *OOMPH – Realistic Holistic Health.* Retrieved from https://www. mondayswholefoods.com/blog/carb-confusion

Foster, H. (2018, 20 May), Is Cell Hacking the Key to Ageing Well? *The Sunday Mail: Body & Soul* [lift out], p. 6.

Frey, M. (2018, 7 February). What are Refined Carbohydrates? *Very Well Fit.* Retrieved from https://www.verywellfit. com/what-are-refined-carbohydrates-3495552

Gaiam. (2016). *A Beginner's Guide to 8 Major Styles of Yoga.* Retrieved from http://www.gaiam.com/discover/167/ article/beginners-guide-8-major-styles-yoga/

Gaudreau, S. (nd). Bone Broth 101: How to Make the Best Bone Broth Recipe. *Stupid Easy Paleo.* Retrieved from https://www.stupideasypaleo.com/2014/07/23/ bone-broth-101-how-to-make-best-broth/

Gebilagin, L. (2017, 14 January). Reach Your Potential: Life Lessons from John Maclean who learned to walk again. *The Daily Telegraph.* Retrieved from http://www.dailytelegraph.com. au/lifestyle/health/body-soul-daily/reach-your-potential- life-lessons-from-john-maclean-who-learned-to-walk-again/ news-story/1076def92fd52a7648ba50213733077c

George Mateljan Foundation, The. (2016), *Turmeric. Retrieved from* http://www.whfoods.com/genpage.php?tname=foodspice& dbid=78

Gerrard, N. (2016, 10 December). A A Gill's Best Lines. *The Caterer.* Retrieved from https://www.thecaterer. com/articles/492920/aa-gills-best-lines

Gerst, A. (2017, 29 May). You Know Saying 'No' Is Important For A Healthy Life. Here's How To Actually Do it. *MindBodyGreen*. Retrieved from https://www.mindbodygreen.com/articles/why-saying-no-is-necessary-for-good-health

Gillespie, D. (2008). *Sweet Poison*, Sydney: Penguin Random House.

Gillett, R. (2017, 28 July). A Japanese Doctor who studied longevity – and lived to be 105 – said if you must retire, do it well after age 65, *Independent*. Retrieved from http://www.independent.co.uk/lifestyle/health-and-families/healthy-living/japanese-doctor-shigeaki-hinohara-st-lukes-international-university-fun-a7864786.html

Glassman, A. (2014, 22 September), How to live to 100 years old as shared by a centenarian. *Chatelaine*. Retrieved from http://www.chatelaine.com/health/how-to-live-to-100-years-old-as-shared-by-a-centenarian/

Gollayan, C. (2018, 23 March). Food-tracking 'tooth Fitbits' are coming for your mouth. *New York Post*. https://nypost.com/2018/03/23/food-tracking-tooth-fitbits-are-coming-for-your-mouth/

Graham, K. (2007). Buddhism and Happiness. *ABC Health & Wellbeing*. Retrieved from http://www.abc.net.au/health/features/stories/2007/10/11/2054844.htm

Graham, L. (2017, 26 February). Is This The New Way To Eat? *Sunday Mail, Body & Soul* [liftout].

Grant, M. (2017, 1 May). Just 10 minutes of meditation helps anxious people have better focus, *Waterloo News*. Retrieved from https://uwaterloo.ca/news/news/just-10-minutes-meditation-helps-anxious-people-have-better

Grattan, L. & Scott, A. (2016). 100-Year Life: Living and Working in an Age of Longevity, London: Bloomsbury.

Graves, G. (2015, 7 May). This Could Be The Simplest Way To Diet Yet—But Do You Have What It Takes To Pull It Off? *Prevention: Health*. Retrieved from https://www.prevention.com/weight-loss/a20456701/simple-fast-to-lose-weight/

Grenville, K. (2017). *The Case Against Fragrance*. Melbourne, Australia: The Text Publishing Company.

Grossman, K. (2018). 10 Reasons to Use Bitters (hint: it all starts with digestive health). *The Radiant Life*. Retrieved from https://blog.radiantlifecatalog.com/bid/70036/10-Reasons-to-Use-Bitters-hint-it-all-starts-with-digestive-health

Group, E. (2014, 23 June). 5 Kidney Cleansing Drinks. *Global Healing Center*, 23 June. Retrieved from https://www.globalhealingcenter.com/natural-health/5-kidney-cleansing-drinks/

Gunnars, K. (2017). 10 Proven Benefits of Green Tea. *Authority Nutrition*. Retrieved from https://authoritynutrition.com/top-10-evidence-based-health-benefits-of-green-tea/

Gupta, S. (2016, 28 April). 6 Benefits of Saving Money. Without Having Extra Money. *Health*. Retrieved from https://www.indiatimes.com/health/healthyliving/6-benefits-of-saving-money-apart-from-having-extra-money-233757.html

Hall, A. (2014, 6 May). The Energy Secret These 15 Successful People Swear By. *HuffPost*. Retrieved from https://www.huffingtonpost.com.au/entry/famous-people-who-nap_n_5248739

Halpern, M. (2015). *Non-Stick, Cast Iron, Or Stainless Steel: Which Is Best?* Retrieved from https://breakingmuscle.com/healthy-eating/non-stick-cast-iron-or-stainless-steel-which-is-best

Hardesty, P. (2016, 6 December). Dive into the Benefits of Swimming. *Huffpost*. Retrieved from https://www.huffingtonpost. com/ornish-living/swimming-benefits_b_8051398.html

Harvard T H Chan School of Public Health. (2018). Healthy Weight: Maintain Don't Gain. *The Nutrition Source*. Retrieved from https://www.hsph.harvard.edu/nutritionsource/healthy-weight/

Harvey, J. (2014, 6 February). Using your breath to improve health and wellbeing. Retrieved from http://head2toehealth.com. au/using-your-breath-to-improve-health-and-wellbeing/

HealthDirect (2016). How to Lower Blood Pressure. Retrieved from http://www.healthdirect.gov.au/how-to-lower-blood-pressure

Healthy Home Economist, The. (2018, 10 January). *Dry Skin Brushing*, 10 January. Retrieved from https://www. thehealthyhomeeconomist.com/dry-skin-brushing-downside/

Heaton, K.W. & Lewis, S.J. (1997). Stool form scale as a useful guide to intestinal transit time. *Scandinavian Journal of Gastroenterology*, Vol.32:9, pp.920-924.

Heid, M. (2015, 11 February). You Asked: Is Perfume Bad for Me? *Time Health*. Retrieved from http://time.com/3703948/ is-perfume-safe/

Hello Sunday Morning. (2018) Retrieved from https://www.hellosundaymorning.org/?utm_ referrer=http%3A%2F%2Fwww.alcohol.gov.au%2Fintern et%2Falcohol%2Fpublishing.nsf%2FContent%2Fhsm

Hellyer, J. (nd). *Lovelife*. Retrieved from http://www.jacqueline hellyer.com/

Hendry, N. (2018). *Dr John Demartini: Saving When Having Credit Card Debts???* [YouTube video-clip]. Retrieved from https://www.youtube.com/watch?v=yhffhGvzv50

Here & Now. (2014, 12 May). *At 99, Anti-Trans Fats Scientist Eats An Egg Daily.* Retrieved from http://www.wbur.org/hereandnow/2014/05/12/trans-fats-scientist

Hill, A. (2017, 13 June). Lion kings: Why cats are the lords of the internet. *The Mercury News.* Retrieved from https://www.mercurynews.com/2017/06/13/lion-kings-why-cats-are-the-lords-of-the-internet/

Ho, V. (2016, August). Potty Talk: Should you Sit your Squat? *LiveScience.* Retrieved from http://www.livescience.com/55777-should-you-sit-or-squat-on-toilet.html

Hobson, R. (2017). Are You Getting Enough Iodine. *Get the Gloss.* Retrieved from https://www.getthegloss.com/article/are-you-getting-enough-iodine

Hodge, A. (2018, 14-15 July). The Great Escape. *The Weekend Australian*, pp. 16-17.

Holt-Lunstad, J., Smith, T.B., Baker, M., Harris. T. & Stephenson., D. (2015, 11 March). Loneliness and Social Isolation as Risk Factors for Mortality: A Meta-Analytic Review. *Perspectives on Psychological Science,* Vol. 10: 2, pp-227-237.

Hooper, J. (2017, 29 October). Is the era of anti-aging over? *The Sunday Mail: Body & Soul* [liftout], p. 4.

Hozer, M. [Director]. (2015). *Sugar Coated* [film]. The Cutting Factory.

Humana. (2014). Pay Attention to Your Poop. Retrieved from https://www.humana.com/learning-center/health-and-wellbeing/healthy-living/feces

Hunter, F. (2018, 6 January). Advertising banned, drinks taxed, vending machines removed: doctors' plan for war on sugar. *The Sydney Morning Herald.* Retrieved from http://www.smh.com.au/federal-politics/political-news/advertising-banned-drinks-taxed-vending-machines-removed-doctors-plan-for-war-on-sugar-20180105-h0duw0.html

Hyman, M. (nd). 10 Reasons to Quit Coffee (Plus Healthy Alternatives). *Hungry for Change.* Retrieved from http://www.hungryforchange.tv/article/10-reasons-to-quit-coffee-plus-healthy-alternatives

IMDB (International Movie Database). (2000), *Pay It Forward* [film]. Retrieved from http://www.imdb.com/title/tt0223897/

IMDB (International Movie Database). (2016, 16 December). *Collateral Beauty* [film]. Retrieved from https://www.imdb.com/title/tt4682786/?ref_=fn_al_tt_1

Indiana University Bloomington. (2015, 16 June). *Not-so-guilty pleasure: Viewing cat videos boosts energy and positive emotions, IU study finds.* Retrieved from http://archive.news.indiana.edu/releases/iu/2015/06/internet-cat-video-research.shtml

Institute for Responsible Nutrition. (2016*). Learn to Recognize the 56 different names for sugar.* Retrieved from http://www.responsiblefoods.org/sugar_names

Internal Gardens Tai Chi. (2012, 27 February). *What Does "Tai Chi Chuan" Mean, and Why is it also Spelled as "Taijiquan?"* Retrieved from http://www.internalgardens.com/does-tai-chi-chuan-mean-why-spelled-as-taijiquan

Islam, S.M., Math, R.K., Cho, K.M., Lim, W.J., Hong, S.Y., Kim J.M., Yun, M.G., Cho, J.J. and Yun, H.D. (2010, 12 May). Organophosphorus hydrolase (OpdB) of Lactobacillus brevis

WCP902 from kimchi is able to degrade organophosphorus pesticides. *Journal of Agriculture and Food Chemistry, ACS Publications*, 58:9, 5380-5386. Retrieved from http://pubs.acs.org/doi/abs/10.1021/jf903878e

James, N. (2017). *10 Strategies for a Digital Detox*. Retrieved from https://neenjames.com/10-strategies-digital-detox/

Jaminet, P. (2010, 18 August). *What Makes a Supercentenarian?* Retrieved from http://perfecthealthdiet. com/2010/08/what-makes-a-supercentenarian/

Jenkins, D. (2017). 10 extra virgin olive oil benefits you never knew. *MyBody+Soul*. Retrieved from http://www.bodyandsoul.com. au/nutrition/nutrition-tips/10-extra-virgin-olive-oil-benefits-you-never-knew/news-story/ea7be0fb323cc7415caec311fd33d576

Johns Hopkins Bloomberg School of Public Health. (2018, 21 February). *Study: Lead and Other Toxic Metals Found in E-Cigarette 'Vapors'.* [Media Release]. Retrieved from https://www.jhsph.edu/news/news-releases/2018/study-lead-and-other-toxic-metals-found-in-e-cigarette-vapors.html

Juan, S. (2006, 10 November). Does Eating Fish Improve Central Nervous System? Oh my, Omega-3. *The Register.* Retrieved from https://www.theregister.co.uk/2006/11/10/the_odd_body_fish_brain_function/

Kallistratos, M. (2015, 29 August). Midday naps associated with reduced blood pressure and fewer medications. *European Society of Cardiology*. Retrieved from https://www.escardio.org/The-ESC/Press-Office/Press-releases/Midday-naps-associated-with-reduced-blood-pressure-and-fewer-medications

Kant, A.K., Andon, T.J. & Angelopoulos, J.M.R. (2008). Association of Breakfast Energy Density with Diet Quality and Body Mass Index in American Adults: National Health and

Nutrition Examination Surveys, 1999-2004. *American Journal of Clinical Nutrition*, 88:5, 1396-1404.

Ketler, A. (2016, 8 May). Here's what happens to your body when you go ten days without sugar. *Collective Evolution*. Retrieved from http://www.collective-evolution.com/2016/05/08/heres-happens-to-your-body-when-you-go-10-days-without-sugar/

King, R. Dr. (2011). *Good Loving Great Sex*. [Kindle Edition]. Australia: RHA eBooks Adult.

King, R. (2017, 5 February). 'Forget Work-Life Balance and Focus on Laughing Every Day Instead'. *The Sunday Mail: Body & Soul* [lift out], p. 4.

King, R. (2017, 14 May). "Music has been an incredible healer for me", *The Sunday Mail: Body & Soul* [lift out], p. 4.

Knapton, S. (2018, 11 March). Knitting should be prescribed on NHS to lower blood pressure, reduce depression and slow dementia. *The Telegraph: Science*. Retrieved from https://www.telegraph.co.uk/science/2018/03/11/knitting-should-prescribed-nhs-lower-blood-pressure-reduce-depression/

Komisaruk, B. (2017). 10 Surprising Health Benefits of Sex. *WebMD*. Retrieved from http://www.webmd.com/sex-relationships/guide/sex-and-health

Kopecky, R. (2016, 20 February). The Awesome Power of the field of Love. *Gaia*. Retrieved from https://www.gaia.com/article/awesome-power-of-the-field-love

Kroeker, A. (2017, 11 October). *Health Benefits of Bone Broth*. Retrieved from https://amykroekernd.com/2017/10/11/health-benefits-of-bone-broth/

Kummerow, F. (2014). Cholesterol is Not the Culprit: A Guide to Preventing Heart Disease, Spacedoc Media, LLC.

Laurie, V. (2018, 18 July). Aussie blood test gets the jump on melanoma. *The Australian*, p. 4.

Lee, C.A., & Clements-Cortes, A. (2014). Applications of clinical improvisation and aesthetic music therapy in medical settings: An analysis of Debussy's 'L'isle joyeuse'. Music and Medicine, 6(2), 61-69. *Research Gate*. Retrieved from https://www.researchgate.net/publication/293178495_Lee_C_A_Clements-Cortes_A_2014_Applications_of_clinical_improvisation_and_aesthetic_music_therapy_in_medical_settings_An_analysis_of_Debussy's_'L'isle_joyeuse'_Music_and_Medicine_62_61-69

Lee, S. (2017, 14 July). Why Indoor Plants Make You Feel Better. *Better*. Retrieved from https://www.nbcnews.com/better/health/indoor-plants-can-instantly-boost-your-health-happiness-ncna781806

Leech, J. (2015, 24 May). 11 Evidence-Based Health Benefits of Eating Fish. *Healthline*. Retrieved from https://www.healthline.com/nutrition/11-health-benefits-of-fish

Lewin, J. (2017). The health benefits of quinoa. *GoodFood*. Retrieved from https://www.bbcgoodfood.com/howto/guide/health-benefits-quinoa

Lighthouse. (2016). "Laughter is the best medicine" – Origin, Meaning, Explanation and Importance. *Important India*. Retrieved from https://www.importantindia.com/23587/laughter-is-the-best-medicine/

Lourie, B. & Smith R. (2010). Slow Death by Rubber Duck: How the Toxic Chemistry of Everyday Life Affects Our Health, Canada: Vintage.

Lourie, B. & Smith R. (2014). *Toxin Toxout,* Brisbane: UQ Press.

Luis, A., Domingues, F. & Pereira, L. (2017, September). Can Cranberries Contribute to Reduce the Incidence of Urinary Tract Infections? A Systematic Review with Meta-Analysis and Trial Sequential Analysis of Clinical Trials. *The Journal of Urology*, 198:3, 614-621, https://www.jurology.com/article/S0022-5347(17)39295-9/abstract

Lustig, R. (2009, 31 July). Sugar: The Bitter Truth. [YouTube]. *University of California Television (UCTV).* Retrieved from https://youtu.be/dBnniua6-oM

Lustig, R. (2012). *Sugar: The Bitter Truth*, CreateSpace Independent Publishing Platform.

Lustig, R. (2013) Sugar Has 56 Names: A Shopper's Guide, Kindle: Avery.

Lustig, R.H., Mulligan, K., Noworolski, S.M., Tai, V. W., Wen, M.J., Erkin-Cakmak, A., Gugliucci, A., Schwarz, J.M. (2016). Isocaloric fructose restriction and metabolic improvement in children with obesity and metabolic syndrome. *Obesity Research Journal*, 24:2, pp. 453-460. Retrieved from http://onlinelibrary.wiley.com/doi/10.1002/oby.21371/abstract

Mackenzie, S. (Editor). (2015). Movement vs. Exercise: Moving out of the (fitness) box. *Best Kept Self*. Retrieved from http://www.bestkeptself.com/2015/03/12/movement-vs-exercise-moving-out-of-the-fitness-box/

MacLellan, L. & Zhou, Y. (2017, 10 June). No Math Required: BMI calculators aren't accurate, but our body fat calculator is. *Quartz.* Retrieved from https://qz.com/1002707/bmi-calculators-arent-accurate-but-our-body-fat-calculator-is/

Makin, S. (2015, 1 September). Feeling Awe May Be Good for Our Health: That thunderstruck feeling is linked to lower inflammation. *Scientific American*. Retrieved from https://www.scientificamerican.com/article/feeling-awe-may-be-good-for-our-health/

Marie, D. (2016, 2 May). Knowledge is power when selected food – and taking control of your health. *Healthy Out Of Habit*. Retrieved from https://www.healthyoutofhabit.com/blog/bittman-vox

Mattson, M.P. (2015). Lifelong brain health is a lifelong challenge: from evolutionary principles to empirical evidence. *Ageing Research,* 20: 37-45 Retrieved from https://www.sciencedirect.com/science/article/pii/S1568163715000021

Mattson, M.P. (2018). The University of Iowa. *College of Liberal Arts and Sciences, Department of Biology.* Retrieved from https://biology.uiowa.edu/alumni/spotlights/mark-mattson

Mayoh, L. (2018, 22 April). Let's Get Flexible. *Sunday Mail: Body & Soul* [liftout], pp. 4-5.

McCall, T. (2007). *38 Health Benefits of Yoga.* Retrieved from http://www.yogajournal.com/article/health/count-yoga-38-ways-yoga-keeps-fit/

McGrath, L. (2017, November). Beetroot – the power behind this superfood, *The House of Wellness.* Retrieved from https://www.houseofwellness.com.au/health/nutrition/beetroot-superfood

McKay, B. (2017, 8 April). Healthy habits to follow if you want to live a long life. *News Limited*. Retrieved from http://www.news.com.au/lifestyle/health/diet/healthy-habits-to-follow-if-you-want-to-live-a-long-life/news-story/3cc70a1f56a2f6d0b8240313536142c1

McMillen, A. (2018, 24 January). Disease Stops Neil Diamond Touring, *The Australian*, p. 3.

Menon, M.K. (2016, 16 January). Advice from the world's oldest marathoner on eating well and living long. *The Indian Express*. Retrieved from https://indianexpress.com/article/lifestyle/fitness/advice-from-the-worlds-oldest-marathoner-on-eating-well-and-living-long/

Mercola, J. (2017). *7 Important Reasons to Properly Chew Your Food*. Retrieved from http://articles.mercola.com/sites/articles/archive/2013/07/31/chewing-foods.aspx

Milliken, B. & Meredith, C. (1968). *Tough Love*, Michigan, USA: Fleming H Revell Company.

Modern Alternative Health. (2017). *Is There Lead In Bentonite Clay?* Retrieved from http://www.modernalternativehealth.com/2014/07/18/lead-bentonite-clay/

MommyPotamus. (2018). *Why Vitamin D3 Supplements May Not Replace Sunshine.* Retrieved from https://www.mommypotamus.com/vitamin-d-supplements/

Morales, K. (2017, 19 April). Skip the caffeine, opt for the stairs to feel more energized. *University of Georgia, UGA Today*. Retrieved from https://news.uga.edu/stairs-more-energy-research/

Moskin, J. (2015, 6 January). Bones, Broth, Bliss: Bone Broth Evolves From Prehistoric Food to Paleo Drink. *The New York Times*. Retrieved from https://www.nytimes.com/2015/01/07/dining/bone-broth-evolves-from-prehistoric-food-to-paleo-drink.html

Moskvitch, K. (2015, 19 November). Can you be too clean? *BBC*, 19 November. retrieved from http://www.bbc.com/future/story/20151118-can-you-be-too-clean

Mosley, M. (2012). *Eat, Fast and Live Longer* [documentary]. Kate Dart [Writer & Director] [52 mins]. Retrieved from http://watchdocumentaries.com/eat-fast-and-live-longer/

Mosley, M. (2015). *The 8-week Blood Sugar Diet.* [Kindle Edition], Australia: Simon & Schuster.

Mosley, M. (2018, 29 January). Why You Need Cow's Milk, *The Australian. Life*, p. 8.

Myers, T. (2015, 27 April). Foam Rolling and Self-Myofascial Release. *Anatomy Trains.* Retrieved from https://www.anatomytrains.com/blog/2015/04/27/foam-rolling-and-self-myofascial-release/

Naeem, Z. (2010, January). Vitamin D Deficiency: An Ignored Epidemic. *International Journal of Health Science.* Retrieved from https://www.ncbi.nlm.nih.gov/pmc/articles/PMC3068797/

National Heart Foundation of Australia. (nd), *Salt.* Retrieved from https://www.heartfoundation.org.au/healthy-eating/food-and-nutrition/salt

NaturalOn. (2018). *Easiest Ways to Detox and Remove Pesticides from Your Body.* Retrieved from https://naturalon.com/easiest-ways-detox-remove-pesticides-body/view-all/

NDTV. (2016, 5 December). *Handful Of Nuts A Day May Cut Heart Disease, Cancer Risk: Study.* Retrieved from https://www.ndtv.com/health/handful-of-nuts-a-day-may-cut-heart-disease-cancer-risk-study-1634072

Newcomer, L. (2017, 23 December). Why you should be eating more bitter foods. *Better.* Retrieved from https://www.nbcnews.com/better/health/why-you-should-be-eating-more-bitter-foods-ncna831091

Nourished Life. (2017). *Is your perfume making you sick?* Retrieved from https://www.nourishedlife.com.au/ article/694642/your-perfume-making-you-sick.html

Nunes, L. (2018). Slow-cooker bone broth. *Taste.com.au.* Retrieved from http://www.taste.com.au/recipes/slow-cooker-bone-broth/a8b0540f-2dc1-45a9-be23-3c442f526b51

Nutrition Australia. (2010, June). *Iodine Facts.* Retrieved from http://www.nutritionaustralia.org/national/resource/iodine-facts

Nuts for Life. (2016, July). *Are Nuts Expensive? Retrieved from* https://www.nutsforlife.com.au/ wp_super_faq/why-are-nuts-so-expensive/

O'Neil, Carol E., Byrd-Bredbenner, C., Hayes, D., Jana, L., Klinger, S.E. & Stephenson-Martin, S. (2014). The Role of Breakfast in Health: Definition and Criteria for a Quality Breakfast. *Journal of the Academy of Nutrition and Dietetics*, 114:12, S8-S26. Retrieved from https:// daa.asn.au/smart-eating-for-you/smart-eating-fast-facts/breakfast-how-to-eat-brekkie-like-a-boss/

O'Neill, D. & Malhotra, A. (2016). *The Big Fat Fix,* [film], Cape Crusaders.

Optometry Australia. (2018). *Your Eye Exam: Medicare.* Retrieved from http://www.optometry.org.au/your-eyes/your-eye-exam/costs/

Optometry Australia. (2018a). *Your Eye Health: UV Protection. Retrieved from* http://www.optometry.org. au/wa/your-eyes/your-eye-health/sun-safety/

Organic Facts. (2017, 14 November). 13 Impressive Benefits of Salt. https://www.organicfacts.net/health-benefits/other/health-benefits-of-salt.html

Osteoporosis Australia. (2012). Vitamin D Consumer guide. Retrieved from https://www.osteoporosis.org.au/sites/default/files/files/vitdconsumerguide.pdf

Padovese, V. (2017, 1 October). The world's top coffee consuming nations – and how they take their cup. *SBS*. Retrieved from https://www.sbs.com.au/yourlanguage/italian/en/article/2017/03/29/worlds-top-coffee-consuming-nations-and-how-they-take-their-cup

Paganini-Hill, A., White, S.C. & Atchison, K.A. (2011, 15 June). Dental Health Behaviours, Dentition, and Mortality in the Elderly: The Leisure World Cohort Study. *Journal of Aging Research.* Retrieved from https://www.ncbi.nlm.nih.gov/pmc/articles/PMC3124861/

Paleo Leap. (2017). *Cooking with Stainless Steel.* Retrieved from https://paleoleap.com/cooking-stainless-steel/

Paleohacks (2014, 19 August). *My house smells horrible with bone broth brewing - am I doing something wrong?* Retrieved from https://www.paleohacks.com/bone-broth/my-house-smells-horrible-with-bone-broth-brewing-am-i-doing-something-wrong-4782

Palermo, E. (2013, 29 July). Do Plants Really Clean the Air? *Live Science.* Retrieved from https://www.livescience.com/38445-indoor-plants-clean-air.html

Pall, M. (2013). Electromagnetic fields act via activation of voltage-gated calcium channels to produce beneficial or adverse effects. *Journal of Cellular and Molecular Medicine*, 17:8, 958-965. Retrieved from http://www.ncbi.nlm.nih.gov/pubmed/23802593

Pall, M. (2014). Microwave electromagnetic fields act by activating voltage-gated calcium channels: why the current international safety standards do not predict biological hazard. *Electromagnetic*

Biological Medicine, 33, p. 251. Retrieved from http://www.
sciencedirect.com/science/article/pii/S0891061815000599

Park, A. (2017, 10 July). Coffee Drinkers Really Do Live
Longer, *Time Health*, 10 July. Retrieved from http://
time.com/4849985/coffee-caffeine-live-longer/

Park, A. (2017, 21 June). How Breastfeeding Lowers a Mom's
Risk of Heart Disease. *Time Health*. Retrieved from http://
time.com/4825665/breastfeeding-heart-benefits/

Park, D.C., Lodi-Smith, J., Drew, L., Haber, S., Hebrank, A.,
Bischof, G.N. & Aamodt, W. (2014). The impact of sustained
engagement on cognitive function in older adults: The
Synapse Project. *Psychological Science*, 25(1), 103-12.

Park, S., Freedman N.D., Haiman, C.A., Le Marchand, L.,
Wilkins, L.R., Setiawan, V.W. (2017, 15 August), Association
of Coffee Consumption With Total and Cause-Specific
Mortality Among Nonwhite Populations. *Annals of Internal
Medicine*. Retrieved from http://annals.org/aim/article-
abstract/2643433/association-coffee-consumption-total-
cause-specific-mortality-among-nonwhite-populations

Passmore, D. (2018, 10 June). Beware the cereal killer,
doctor says, *The Sunday Mail*: News, p. 31.

Peat, R. (2015, 18 December). 101 Year Old Fred Kummerow Exercised
A Lot And Eats Whole Grains, Oatmeal, And Vegetables.
Perceive Think Act. Retrieved from https://raypeatforum.com/
community/threads/101-year-old-fred-kummerow-exercised-
a-lot-and-eats-whole-grains-oatmeal-and-vegetables.8933/

Peeling, P. (2016, 7 March). Can beetroot juice give elite athletes an
edge? *The University of Western Australia:* University News.
Retrieved from http://www.news.uwa.edu.au/201603078412/
research/can-beetroot-juice-give-elite-athletes-edge

Petrucci, K. (2016). *Why Collagen Bone Broth is Liquid Gold*. [YouTube Video clip]. Retrieved from https://www.youtube.com/watch?v=OBv4SmMyDfQ

Petrucci, K. (2017). *Do You Suffer From Histamine Intolerance?* Retrieved from https://www.drkellyann.com/do-you-suffer-from-histamine-intolerance/

Pie, J. (2016). Adaptogen Herbs: Nature's Stress and Fatigue Fighters. *Changing Habits*. Retrieved from https://changinghabits.com.au/adaptogen-herbs-natures-stress-and-fatigue-fighters/

Piff, P.K., Dietz, P., Feinberg, M., Sancato, D.M. & Keltner, D. (2015). Awe, the Small Self, and Prosocial Behavior. *Journal of Personality and Social Psychology*, 108:6, 883-899. Retrieved from http://www.apa.org/pubs/journals/releases/psp-pspi0000018.pdf

Pioneer Woman, The. (2017). *How to Make Ghee*. Retrieved from http://thepioneerwoman.com/food-and-friends/how-to-make-ghee/

Pitt, T. & Corbett, B. (2018). *Unmasked*, North Sydney, Australia: Penguin Random House Australia.

Potter, C. (2013, 12 August). Stretches for your calf, quadricep, hamstring, chest, shoulder and tricep. *BUPA Health UK*. Retrieved from https://www.youtube.com/watch?v=WnZ8snlfNec

Powell, S. (2018, 29 May). Smoking Without Guilt, *The Australian*: Inquirer, p. 11.

PRD Enterprises. (2012). *The Acid & Alkaline pH Chart*. Retrieved from http://www.booktopia.com.au/the-acid-alkaline-ph-chart-prd-enterprises/prod0609613826412.html

Proactive Health. (nd). *Green Homes Bathroom Pocket Guide*. Retrieved from http://www. proactivehealth.net.au/index.php?mp_id=5

Puterbaugh, P. (1985, 9 May), A Sense of Wonder. *Rolling Stone*. Retrieved from https://www.rollingstone.com/music/ music-album-reviews/a-sense-of-wonder-93506/

Queensland Health, Oral Health Unit. (2017). *Healthy Teeth for Life*. Retrieved from https://www.health.qld.gov.au/oralhealth

Quigley, G. (2017, October). A Word of Advice: COQ10 retards various aspects of the ageing process, including within the brain. *The House of Wellness*, p. 5.

QuitNow, Australian Government. (2017, 6 December). *How Smoking Damages Your Body*. Retrieved from https://ww.quitnow.gov.au

Raloff, J. (2016, 12 February). Vaping linked to host of new health risks. *Science News*. Retrieved from https://www.sciencenews.org

Rehfeld, K., Müller, P., Aye, N., Schmicker, M., Dordevic, M., Kaufmann, J., Hökelmann, A. and Müller, N.G. (2017, 15 June). Dancing or Fitness Sport? The Effects of Two Training Programs on Hippocampal Plasticity and Balance Abilities in Healthy Seniors. *Frontier Human Neuroscience*, 11:305. Retrieved from https://www. frontiersin.org/articles/10.3389/fnhum.2017.00305/full

Rehme, M.G. (2005). *How a Dentist Can Save Your Life*. Retrieved from http://toothbody.com/how-your-dentist-can-save-your-life/

Rhodes, J. (2015, 13 September). Top 25 Mentoring Relationships in History. *The Chronicle of Evidence-Based Mentoring*. Retrieved from https://chronicle.umbmentoring. org/top-25-mentoring-relationships-in-history/

Ringland, J. (2017, 22 January). Why Having a Pet Makes Life Better, *The Sunday Mail*: *Body+Soul* [liftout], p. 4.

Robbins, A. (2012). *What do you really want in life? Retrieved from* https://www.youtube.com/watch?v=H0guq15_S4E

Robinson, L., Smith, M.A. & Segal, J. (2017). Laughter is the Best Medicine: The Health Benefits of Humor and Laughter. *Helpguide.org. Retrieved from* https://www.helpguide.org/articles/mental-health/laughter-is-the-best-medicine.htm

Robinson, M.M., Dasari, S., Konopka, A.R., Johnson, M.L., Manjunatha, S., Esponda, R.R., Carter, R.E., Lanza, I.R. & Nair, K.S. (2017, 7 March). Enhanced Protein Translation Underlies Improved Metabolic and Physical Adaptations to Different Exercise Training Modes in Young and Old Humans. *Cell Metabolism*, 25:3, 581-592 Retrieved from https://www.cell.com/cell-metabolism/fulltext/S1550-4131(17)30099-2

Rodie, C. (2017, 19 February). Roll Your Way to Better Health, *The Sunday Mail*: *Body+Soul* [Liftout], pp.10-11.

Romundstad, S., Svebak, S., Holen, A. & Holmen, J. (2016). A 15-Year Follow-Up Study of Sense of Humor and Causes of Mortality: The Nord-Trøndelag Health Study. *Psychomatic Medicine*, 78:3, 345-353. Retrieved from https://journals.lww.com/psychosomaticmedicine/Abstract/2016/04000/A_15_Year_Follow_Up_Study_of_Sense_of_Humor_and.12.aspx

Royal Society for the Prevention of Cruelty to Animals (RSPCA). (2015). *What are the Health Benefits of Pet Ownership?* Retrieved from http://kb.rspca.org.au/what-are-the-health-benefits-of-pet-ownership_408.html

Sachdev, P. (2013, June). The Sydney Centenarian Study: methodology and profile of centenarians and near-centenarians. *International Psychogeriatrics*, 25:6, 99-1005.

Salehi, A., Hashemi, N., Imanieh, M.H. & Saber, M. (2015, October). Chiropractic: Is it Efficient in Treatment of Diseases? Review of Systematic Reviews. *International Journal of Community Based Nursing and Midwifery,* 3(4): 244-254. Retrieved from https://www.ncbi.nlm.nih.gov/pmc/articles/PMC4591574/

Samadi, D. (2017, 6 January). Sugar Is Not Only a Drug but a Poison Too. *Life.* Retrieved from https://www.huffpost.com/entry/sugar-is-not-only-a-drug-but-a-poison-too_b_8918630

Sass, C. (2015, 27 March). 7 Things You Should Know About Matcha. *Health.* Retrieved from http://www.health.com/nutrition/what-is-matcha

Schlitz, M. (2017), The Grateful Aging Program: A Naturalistic Model of Transformation and Healing into the Second Half of Life. *The Permanente Journal: US National Library of Medicine,* 21: 16-82. Retrieved from https://www.ncbi.nlm.nih.gov/pmc/articles/PMC5283784/

Second Opinion. (2016). *Longevity: Aging.* Episode 311. Retrieved from https://www.secondopinion-tv.org/episode/longevity

Seiga-Riz, A.M., Popkin, B.M. & Carson T. (1998). Trends in breakfast consumption for children in the United States from 1965 – 1991. *American Journal of Clinical Nutrition,* 67:4, 748S-756S. Retrieved from https://www.ncbi.nlm.nih.gov/pubmed/9537624

Selhub, E.M., Logan, A.L & Bested, A.C. (2014, 15 January). Fermented foods, microbiota, and mental health: ancient practice meets nutritional psychiatry. *Journal of Physiological Anthropology,* 33:2. Retrieved from https://doi.org/10.1186/1880-6805-33-2

Shah, Y. (2016, 23 February). Badass 110-Year-Old Birthday Girl Loves Naps, Hates TV Crews. *HuffPost.* Retrieved from https://www.

huffingtonpost.com.au/entry/badass-110-year-old-birthday-girl-loves-naps-hates-tv-crews_us_56cb25c1e4b041136f178d0c

Shakespeare, W. (2006). *All's Well That Ends Well.* Barbara A. Mowat (Ed.) Folger Shakespeare Library, 1st Edition, IV, 3, 80. New York: Simon & Shuster.

Sharman, L & Dingle, G.A. (2015, 21 May). Extreme metal music and anger processing. *Frontiers in Human Neuroscience.* Retrieved from http://journal.frontiersin.org/article/10.3389/fnhum.2015.00272/full

Shea, G.F. (1997). *Mentoring* (Rev. Ed.). Menlo Park, California: Crisp Publications. Retrieved from http://www.learningservices.emory.edu/mentor_emory/mentorstory.html

Shecter, A., Kim, W.K., St-Onge, M.P. & Westwood, A.J. (2018, January). Blocking nocturnal blue light for insomnia: A randomized controlled trial. *Journal of Psychiatric Research*, January, 96: 196-202. Retrieved from https://www.journalofpsychiatricresearch.com/article/S0022-3956(17)30859-2/abstract

Shipard, I. (2003), How Can I Use Herbs in my Daily Life?: Over 500 herbs, spices and edible plants: an Australian practical guide to growing, with culinary and medicinal uses, (6th edition). David Stewart: Nambour, Australia.

Sifferlin, A. (2013, 2 April). Fish: The Fountain of Youth? *Time Heart Disease.* http://healthland.time.com/2013/04/02/fish-the-fountain-of-youth

Sifferlin, A. (2016, 15 July). When to Eat Breakfast, Lunch and Dinner. *Time Health.* Retrieved from http://time.com/4408772/best-times-breakfast-lunch-dinner/

Sifferlin, A. (2018, 9 March). How Exercising Into Old Age Can Keep Your Immune System Young. *Time Health.* Retrieved from http://time.com/5193032/cycling-old-age-immune-system/

Sigley, P. (2018, 8 May). The Secret to Longevity according to a Study of Centenarians. *The Sydney Morning Herald: Lifestyle.* Retrieved from https://www.smh.com.au/lifestyle/health-and-wellness/the-secret-to-longevity-according-to-a-study-of-centenarians-20180508-p4ze1x.html

Sisson, M. (2011). Mark's Daily Apple - Earthing: Another Reason to go barefoot. Retrieved from http://www.marksdailyapple.com/earthing/#ixzz48Jwkr79E

Sisson, M. (2013). The Primal Connection: Follow your Genetic Blueprint to Health and Happiness. Primal Nutrition Inc.

Snodgrass, E. (2013, 25 October). Tomb of Ancient Physician Discovered. *National Geographic.* Retrieved from https://news.nationalgeographic.com/news/2013/10/131025-tomb-abusir-discovery-physician-ancient-egypt-archaeology-science/

Spector, T. (2016, 4 July). Most of what we eat is 'processed' food. Here's why we should be worried. *Diet and Fitness.* Retrieved from http://health.spectator.co.uk/most-of-what-we-eat-is-processed-food-heres-why-we-should-be- worried/?utm_medium=social&utm_source=twitter

Spencer, B. (2017). DON'T skip breakfast! Official advice warns that missing out on a morning meal raises the risk of obesity, heart disease and diabetes. *Daily Mail.* Retrieved from http://www.dailymail.co.uk/health/article-4172850/DON-T-skip-breakfast.html

Spinks, R. (2018, 20 February). Britain's tea habit has a plastic problem. *Quartzy.* Retrieved from https://quartzy.qz.com/1210650/most-of-britains-tea-bags-contain-plastic/

Spiritual Cinema Circle. (2015). *Kindness is Contagious.*[DVD], Vol. 12.

Spritzler, F. (2016, 13 July). 8 Signs and Symptoms of Vitamin D Deficiency. *Healthline.* Retrieved from https://www. healthline.com/nutrition/vitamin-d-deficiency-symptoms

Squatty Potty. (2018). Retrieved from http://www. squattypottyaustralia.com/?gclid=EAIaIQobChMI3JTv tYva3QIVzbftCh32FAaOEAAYASAAEgI2GvD_BwE

Stanaway, F.F., Gnjidic, D., Blyth F.M., Le Couteur, D.G., Naganathan, V., Waite. L., Seibel, M.J., Handelsman, D.J., Sambrook, P.N. & Cumming, R.G. (2011, 15 December). How fast does the Grim Reaper walk? Receiver operating characteristics curve analysis in healthy men aged 70 and over. *BMJ,* 343:1-4, https://www.ncbi.nlm.nih.gov/pubmed/22174324

Statista. (2018). *Number of Smartphone Users worldwide from 2014 to 2020 (in billions).* Retrieved from https://www.statista.com/ statistics/330695/number-of-smartphone-users-worldwide/

Statistics Finland. (2015). *Causes of death in 2015.* Retrieved from https://www.stat.fi/til/ksyyt/2015/ ksyyt_2015_2016-12-30_kat_001_en.html

Steber, C. (2018, 13 January). 11 Surprising Health Effects Of Taking Long Showers. *Bustle.* Retrieved from https://www.bustle.com/ p/11-surprising-health-effects-of-taking-long-showers-7844515

Stephenson, K. (2016, 22 October). Faecal transplants: 'My dad's poo saved my life'. *Daily Telegraph.* Retrieved from https://www.dailytelegraph.com.au/lifestyle/ health/body-soul-daily/faecal-transplants-can-restore-health--soon-we-might-be-popping-crapsules/news-story/7c91f280dcd8954d06d720acfbef8721

Strauss-Blasche G., Ekmekcioglu C., & Marktl W. (2000, April). Does vacation enable recuperation? Changes in wellbeing associated with time away from work. *Occupational Medicine*. 50(3), 167-72. Retrieved from https://www.ncbi.nlm.nih.gov/pubmed/10912359

Streicher, L. (2013). 10 Surprising Health Benefits of Sex. *WebMD*. Retrieved from http://www.webmd.com/sex-relationships/guide/sex-and-health

Sugarman, J. (2016, Spring/Summer). Are There Any Proven Benefits to Fasting? *Johns Hopkins Health Review,* 3:1. Retrieved from http://www.johnshopkinshealthreview.com/issues/spring-summer-2016/articles/are-there-any-proven-benefits-to-fasting

Sveinbjornsdottir, S. (2016, 11 July). The clinical symptoms of Parkinson's disease. *Journal of Neurochemistry*. 139, 318–324.

Tergesen, A. (2015, 23 October). Learn to Love Growing Old. *The Weekend Australian: Health & Wellbeing*. Retrieved from https://www.theaustralian.com.au/life/health-wellbeing/learn-to-love-growing-old/news-story/b2643de877f28968fc390ce6b65407ae

Timlin, M.T., Pereira, M.A., Story, M. & Neumark-Sztainer, D. (2008, March). Breakfast Eating and Weight Change in a 5-Year Prospective Analysis of Adolescents: Project EAT (Eating Among Teens). *American Academy of Paediatrics,* 121:3, e638-e645. Retrieved from http://pediatrics.aappublications.org/content/121/3/e638.short

To Lower Blood Pressure. (2012). Retrieved from http://www.tolowerbloodpressure.com/2012/01/drink-water-benefits-and-interest.html

Tremendous Leadership. (2018). *Charlie (Tremendous) Jones 1927-2008*. https://tremendousleadership.com/pages/charlie

United States Environmental Protection Agency.
(2017). *Learn about Lead*. Retrieved from https://
www.epa.gov/lead/learn-about-lead

University of Sydney, The. (2016, 25 October). Increasing
muscle strength can improve brain function: study.
News. Retrieved from https://sydney.edu.au/news-
opinion/news/2016/10/25/increasing-muscle-
strength-can-improve-brain-function--study.html

Van den Berg, L. (2018, 23 May). Diet Key to
Mood Swings, *The Courier-Mail*, p. 7.

Verge, The. (2018, 4 June). Apple WWDC2018 in 14 minutes.
Retrieved from https://www.youtube.com/watch?v=CORL6kACgE4

Vitamin D Council. (2017, 4 May). *Review establishes vitamin D
deficiency risk factors, prevalence and treatment for individuals
worldwide*. Retrieved from https://www.vitamindcouncil.
org/review-establishes-vitamin-d-deficiency-risk-factors-
prevalence-and-treatment-for-individuals-worldwide/

Wagland, B. (nd). Integrating Mind, Body and Spirit through Tai
Chi. *Tai Chi Academy, Tai Chi for Life*. Retrieved from https://
www.taichiacademy.com.au/magazine/feature53.htm

Walker, M. (2017). Why We Sleep: The New Science of
Sleep and Dreams, London: Penguin Books Ltd.

Wansink, B., & Ittersum, K.V. (2012). Fast Food Restaurant
Lighting and Music Can Reduce Calorie Intake and
Increase Satisfaction. *Psychological Reports: Human
Resources & Marketing*, 111(1), 1-5. Retrieved from http://
foodpsychology.cornell.edu/discoveries/music-and-light

Watson, S. (2013, 26 June). Volunteering may be good for
body and mind. *Harvard Health Publishing*. Retrieved

from https://www.health.harvard.edu/blog/volunteering-may-be-good-for-body-and-mind-201306266428

Watts, K. (2017). 6 Surprising Benefits of Massage Therapy. *Reader's Digest Best Health*. Retrieved from http://www.besthealthmag.ca/best-you/health/benefits-of-massage-therapy/

Weaver, L. (2013). *Beauty From The Inside Out.* China: Little Green Frog Publishing.

Weaver, L. (2015), *Exhausted to Energised*. China: Little Green Frog Publishing.

Weaver, L. (2016a, November). Daily Habits to keep your gut healthy. *Dr Libby*: Newsletter. Retrieved from https://www.drlibby.com/nutrition/daily-habits-help-keep-gut-healthy/#australia

Weaver, L. (2016b). Dr Libby's Women's Wellness Wisdom: What Every Woman Needs To Know, China: Little Green Frog Publishing.

Weaver, L. (2017, 16 May). Dr Libby: The importance of building muscle. *Well&Good*. Retrieved from https://www.stuff.co.nz/life-style/well-good/motivate-me/92522876/dr-libby-the-importance-of-building-muscle

Weaver, L. (nd), The Impact of Alcohol. *Dr Libby*. Retrieved from https://www.drlibby.com/health-wellbeing/the-impact-of-alcohol/

WebMD. (nd). *How to Quit Smoking*. Retrieved from https://www.webmd.com/smoking-cessation/quit-smoking#1

Webster, L. (2018, 29 April). Should sugar be classified in the same category as heroin? *The Hill*. Retrieved from http://thehill.com/opinion/healthcare/385376-should-sugar-be-classified-in-the-same-category-as-heroin

Wedeman, B. (2016, 19 October). How to live to 100: Town full of centenarians spills its secrets, *CNN: Health.* Retrieved from https://edition.cnn.com/2016/09/21/health/how-to-live-to-100-acciaroli-centenarians/index.html

Wellness Mama. (2017). *The Benefits of Bentonite Clay.* Retrieved from https://wellnessmama.com/5915/bentonite-clay-benefits/

Wellness Mama. (2017a). *Remineralizing Tooth Powder Recipe.* Retrieved from https://wellnessmama.com/5252/remineralizing-tooth-powder/

Westcott, W.L. (2012). Resistance training is medicine: effects of strength training on health. *Current Sports Medicine Reports,* 11(4), 209-216. Retrieved from https://www.ncbi.nlm.nih.gov/pubmed/22777332

Westerdal, M. (2018, 11 March). Unlock Your Hip Flexors Mike Westerdal - Best Way to Unlock Hip Flexors. Retrieved from https://www.youtube.com/watch?v=T_GX_KagTMg

White, C. (2017, 17 May). Is 10,000 steps a day enough to keep you healthy? *ABC Health & Wellbeing.* Retrieved from http://www.abc.net.au/news/health/2017-05-17/10000-steps-is-it-enough/8532768

Whiteman, H. (2017, 6 May). Massaging your partner can boost your wellbeing, reduce stress. *MedicalNewsToday.* Retrieved from https://www.medicalnewstoday.com/articles/317315.php

Wilderness Chiropractic Health and Wellness Center. (2012). *Mechanism vs vitalism.* Retrieved from http://wildernesschiropractic.com/mechanism-vs-vitalism/

Wilken, R., Veena, M.S., Wang, M.B. & Srivastan, E.S. (2011, February 7), Curcumin: A review of anti-cancer properties and therapeutic activity in head and neck squamous cell carcinoma. *Molecular Cancer, 10:12*. Retrieved from https://www.ncbi.nlm.nih.gov/pmc/articles/PMC3055228/Willcox, C., Willcox, B.J., Todoriki, H. & Suzuki, M. (2009, August). The Okinawan Diet: Health Implications of a Low-Calorie, Nutrient-Dense, Antioxidant-Rich Dietary Pattern Low in Glycemic Load. *Journal of the American College of Nutrition*. Retrieved from https://www.ncbi.nlm.nih.gov/pubmed/20234038

Williams, S. (2013, 11 August). The 10 Most Common Reasons People Visit Their Doctor. *The Motely Fool*. Retrieved from https://www.fool.com/investing/general/2013/08/11/the-10-most-common-reasons-people-visit-their-doct.aspx

Wolfe, D. (2016). *Drink Water First Thing in the Morning for These 5 Reasons*! Retrieved from https://www.davidwolfe.com/drink-water-first-morning-5-reasons/

Wormer, E.J. (1999, March). A taste for salt in the history of medicine. *Science Tribune*. Retrieved from https://www.tribunes.com/tribune/sel/worm.htm

Wylde, S. (2017). Moving Stretch: Work Your Fascia to Free Your Body. *Amazon Digital Services* [Kindle]. North Atlantic Books.

Wyndham, R. (2014). Dry Body Brush. *Dr. Rach*. Retrieved from http://drrachelwyndham.com/dry-body-brush/

Xtend Life. (2011, August). *Cycling Themselves Into Early Graves….* Retrieved from https://au.xtend-life.com/blogs/health-articles/cycling-themselves-into-early-graves

Yabsley, C. (2017, 8 October). Tired? Anxious? Brain Fog? It Might Be Time To Check Your Copper. *The Sunday Mail: Body+Soul*, 4-5.

Yeager, S. (2018, 29August). The Best High-Intensity Interval-Training Workouts for Cyclist. *Bicycling*. Retrieved from https://www.bicycling.com/training/a20045510/the-best-high-intensity-interval-training-workouts-for-cyclists/

Young, A. (2018, 12 January). 6 Things That Happened When I Tried Intermittent Fasting For A Week, *Prevention: Health*. Retrieved from https://www.prevention.com/food-nutrition/a20478171/i-tried-intermittent-fasting-for-a-week/

Yudkin, J. (1972). Pure, White and Deadly: The Problem of Sugar. London: Davis-Poynter.

Zijian, L. (2016). *The Yangtze Great Chivalrous Man*. Retrieved from https://luzijian.com/

Zimmermann, J., & Neyer, F. J. (2013). Do we become a different person when hitting the road? Personality development of sojourners. *Journal of Personality and Social Psychology, 105*(3), 515-530. Retrieved from http://dx.doi.org/10.1037/a0033019